Fast Facts for the NEW NURSE PRACTITIONER: Wha* ʸ   ed to
Know in a Nutshell, 2e (Aktan)

Fast Facts for the ER NURSE·   ell,
2e (Buettner)

Fast Facts for the MEDICAL-   a
Nutshell (Ciocco)

Fast Facts for the NURSE PRI
Preceptorship in a Nutshell (Ci⟨

Fast Facts for the OPERATING   Orientation and Care Guide
in a Nutshell (Criscitelli)

Fast Facts for the ANTEPARTUM AND POSTPARTUM NURSE: A Nursing
Orientation and Care Guide in a Nutshell (Davidson)

Fast Facts for the NEONATAL NURSE: A Nursing Orientation and Care Guide in
a Nutshell (Davidson)

Fast Facts About PRESSURE ULCER CARE FOR NURSES: How to Prevent,
Detect, and Resolve Them in a Nutshell (Dziedzic)

Fast Facts for the GERONTOLOGY NURSE: A Nursing Care Guide
in a Nutshell (Eliopoulos)

Fast Facts for the LONG-TERM CARE NURSE: What Nursing Home and
Assisted Living Nurses Need to Know in a Nutshell (Eliopoulos)

Fast Facts for the CLINICAL NURSE MANAGER: Managing a Changing
Workplace in a Nutshell, 2e (Fry)

Fast Facts for EVIDENCE-BASED PRACTICE: Implementing EBP in
a Nutshell, 2e (Godshall)

Fast Facts About NURSING AND THE LAW: Law for Nurses in a Nutshell
(Grant, Ballard)

Fast Facts for the L&D NURSE: Labor & Delivery Orientation in a Nutshell, 2e
(Groll)

Fast Facts for the RADIOLOGY NURSE: An Orientation and Nursing Care Guide
in a Nutshell (Grossman)

**Fast Facts on ADOLESCENT HEALTH FOR NURSING AND HEALTH
PROFESSIONALS:** A Care Guide in a Nutshell (Herrman)

Fast Facts for the FAITH COMMUNITY NURSE: Implementing FCN/Parish
Nursing in a Nutshell (Hickman)

Fast Facts for the CARDIAC SURGERY NURSE: Caring for Cardiac Surgery
Patients in a Nutshell, 2e (Hodge)

Fast Facts for the CLINICAL NURSING INSTRUCTOR: Clinical Teaching
in a Nutshell, 2e (Kan, Stabler-Haas)

Fast Facts for the WOUND CARE NURSE: Practical Wound Management
in a Nutshell (Kifer)

Fast Facts About EKGs FOR NURSES: The Rules of Identifying EKGs
in a Nutshell (Landrum)

Fast Facts for the CRITICAL CARE NURSE: Critical Care Nursing
in a Nutshell (Landrum)

Fast Facts for the TRAVEL NURSE: Travel Nursing in a Nutshell (Landrum)

Fast Facts for the SCHOOL NURSE: School Nursing in a Nutshell, 2e (Loschiavo)

Fast Facts About CURRICULUM DEVELOPMENT IN NURSING: How to Develop &
Evaluate Educational Programs in a Nutshell (McCoy, Anema)

Fast Facts for DEMENTIA CARE: What Nurses Need to Know in a Nutshell (Miller)

Fast Facts for HEALTH PROMOTION IN NURSING: *Promoting Wellness in a Nutshell* (Miller)

Fast Facts for STROKE CARE NURSING: *An Expert Guide in a Nutshell* (Morrison)

Fast Facts for the MEDICAL OFFICE NURSE: *What You Really Need to Know in a Nutshell* (Richmeier)

Fast Facts for the PEDIATRIC NURSE: *An Orientation Guide in a Nutshell* (Rupert, Young)

Fast Facts About the GYNECOLOGICAL EXAM FOR NURSE PRACTITIONERS: *Conducting the GYN Exam in a Nutshell* (Secor, Fantasia)

Fast Facts for the STUDENT NURSE: *Nursing Student Success in a Nutshell* (Stabler-Haas)

Fast Facts for CAREER SUCCESS IN NURSING: *Making the Most of Mentoring in a Nutshell* (Vance)

Fast Facts for the TRIAGE NURSE: *An Orientation and Care Guide in a Nutshell* (Visser, Montejano, Grossman)

Fast Facts for DEVELOPING A NURSING ACADEMIC PORTFOLIO: *What You Really Need to Know in a Nutshell* (Wittmann-Price)

Fast Facts for the CLASSROOM NURSING INSTRUCTOR: *Classroom Teaching in a Nutshell* (Yoder-Wise, Kowalski)

Forthcoming FAST FACTS Books

Fast Facts for TESTING AND EVALUATION IN NURSING: *Teaching Skills in a Nutshell* (Dusaj)

Fast Facts About the NURSING PROFESSION: *Historical Perspectives in a Nutshell* (Hunt)

Fast Facts for the HOSPICE NURSE: *A Concise Guide to End-of-Life Care* (Wright)

Visit www.springerpub.com to order.

FAST FACTS FOR THE TRIAGE NURSE

Lynn Sayre Visser, MSN, BS, RN, CEN, CPEN, CLNC, is a registered nurse with more than two decades of experience, including work in pre-hospital care, emergency department (ED), intensive care unit, post-anesthesia recovery, and organ procurement settings. She is a gifted triage educator and has been instrumental in a number of front-end process improvement projects including the implementation of a medical provider in the triage area. Mrs. Visser's involvement in the advancement of triage education, triage practice, and quality patient care earned her, along with Mrs. Montejano, a nomination for the Emergency Nurses Association Team Award. Her professional scholarship includes 20 years of membership in Sigma Theta Tau International, the Honor Society of Nursing, along with contributions to journal articles, book chapters, blogs, and learning modules, both as an author and as a reviewer. She co-authored "What is a Triage Nurse?" published in the *Journal of Emergency Nursing* and is the author of "On the Other Side of the Rails" in the *Journal of Radiology Nursing*. Her involvement with the Emergency Nurses Association includes the honors of being the 2011 national conference blogger, an EMINENCE program mentee, two-time academic scholarship recipient, and a conference poster presenter.

Anna Sivo Montejano, MSN Ed, RN, CEN, has 30 years of experience in emergency nursing and triage education. She has taught nursing theory and aided the professional development of nurses as a preceptor, mentor, and clinical instructor. She has been a certified emergency nurse for more than 25 years. Her ED contributions include work as a staff nurse, primary preceptor, and assistant nurse manager, as well as in educational development. Mrs. Montejano has worked to improve the quality and efficiency of patient care through projects such as the change process of rapid medical screenings and rapid triage assessments, as a project manager for a major ED expansion, and as an advanced cardiac life support instructor. She co-authored "What Is a Triage Nurse?" published in the *Journal of Emergency Nursing*. She is the recipient, along with Mrs. Visser, of a nomination for the Emergency Nurses Association Team Award for her involvement with improvements in triage processes. She received her master's degree in nursing with a focus on education from the University of Phoenix, and her bachelor of science in nursing from California State University, Fresno.

Valerie Aarne Grossman, BSN, RN, MALS, NE-BC, is a registered nurse with more than three decades of diverse nursing experience, including direct patient care, hospital leadership, professional service, and writing for publication. She has worked in a variety of settings, including ED, telephone triage, radiology, and administration. She has volunteered her service to such groups as the Emergency Nurses Association, the Association of Radiology and Imaging Nurses, RAD-AID.org, and the National Certification Corporation, as well as serving on the Research Subject Review Board at the University of Rochester, the New York State Board for Nursing, and SCORE Board (Stakeholders for Care in Oncology and Research for the Elderly). She serves on the editorial boards for the *Journal of Hospital Administration* and the *Journal of Radiology Nursing*, as well as the international advisory board for the journal *Nurse Education Today*. She is the author of numerous peer-reviewed journal articles, chapters, and books, including the *Quick Reference to Triage* and *Emergency Nursing: 5 Tier Triage*. She has been named the 2016 Radiology Nurse of the Year by the Association for Radiologic and Imaging Nursing, which is the association's highest award given in recognition of outstanding radiology nursing practice as demonstrated through leadership, mentorship, and ongoing professional development.

Contributors

Shelley Cohen, MSN, RN, CEN
Educator/Consultant
Health Resources Unlimited
Staff Nurse
Williamson Medical Center
Franklin, Tennessee

Dawn Friedly Gray, MSN, RN, CEN, CCRN
Clinical Coordinator
Emergency Department
Paoli Hospital
Paoli, Pennsylvania

Reneé Semonin Holleran, PhD, FNP-BC, CEN, CCRN (alumnus), CFRN and CTRN (retired), FAEN, Former Editor-in-Chief of the *Journal of Emergency Nursing* (2006–2013)
Nurse Practitioner
Alta View Senior Clinic
Hope Free Clinic
Salt Lake City, Utah

Deb Jeffries, MSN Ed, RN-BC, CEN, CPEN
Clinical Education Specialist
Banner Desert Medical Center
Emergency Department
Cardon Children's Medical Center Emergency Department
Mesa, Arizona

Rebecca S. McNair, RN, CEN
President/Founder
Triage First, Inc.
Fairview, North Carolina

Polly Gerber Zimmermann, MS, MBA, RN, CEN, FAEN
Associate Professor
Harry S Truman College
Chicago, Illinois

FAST FACTS FOR THE TRIAGE NURSE

An Orientation and Care Guide in a Nutshell

Lynn Sayre Visser, MSN, BS, RN, CEN, CPEN, CLNC

Anna Sivo Montejano, MSN Ed, RN, CEN

Valerie Aarne Grossman, BSN, RN, MALS, NE-BC

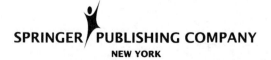

SPRINGER PUBLISHING COMPANY
NEW YORK

PENSACOLA STATE-WAR LIBRARY

Copyright © 2015 Springer Publishing Company, LLC

All rights reserved.

No part of this publication may be reproduced, stored in a retrieval system, or transmitted in any form or by any means, electronic, mechanical, photocopying, recording, or otherwise, without the prior permission of Springer Publishing Company, LLC, or authorization through payment of the appropriate fees to the Copyright Clearance Center, Inc., 222 Rosewood Drive, Danvers, MA 01923, 978-750-8400, fax 978-646-8600, info@copyright.com or on the Web at www.copyright.com.

Springer Publishing Company, LLC
11 West 42nd Street
New York, NY 10036
www.springerpub.com

Acquisitions Editor: Elizabeth Nieginski
Production Editor: Kris Parrish
Composition: S4Carlisle Publishing Services

ISBN: 978-0-8261-2265-0
e-book ISBN: 978-0-8261-2266-7

16 17 18 / 5 4 3 2

The author and the publisher of this Work have made every effort to use sources believed to be reliable to provide information that is accurate and compatible with the standards generally accepted at the time of publication. Because medical science is continually advancing, our knowledge base continues to expand. Therefore, as new information becomes available, changes in procedures become necessary. We recommend that the reader always consult current research and specific institutional policies before performing any clinical procedure. The author and publisher shall not be liable for any special, consequential, or exemplary damages resulting, in whole or in part, from the readers' use of, or reliance on, the information contained in this book. The publisher has no responsibility for the persistence or accuracy of URLs for external or third-party Internet websites referred to in this publication and does not guarantee that any content on such websites is, or will remain, accurate or appropriate.

Library of Congress Cataloging-in-Publication Data

Fast facts for the triage nurse : an orientation and care guide in a nutshell / [edited by] Lynn Sayre Visser, Anna Sivo Montejano, Valerie Aarne Grossman.
     p. ; cm.—(Fast facts)
  Includes bibliographical references and index.
  ISBN 978-0-8261-2265-0—ISBN 978-0-8261-2266-7 (e-book)
  I. Visser, Lynn Sayre, editor. II. Montejano, Anna Sivo, editor. III. Grossman, Valerie Aarne, editor. IV. Series: Fast facts (Springer Publishing Company)
  [DNLM: 1. Emergencies—nursing. 2. Triage—methods. 3. Emergency Nursing—methods. 4. Emergency Treatment—nursing WY 154.2]
  RC86.7
  616.02'5—dc23
                                                                              2015004961

Special discounts on bulk quantities of our books are available to corporations, professional associations, pharmaceutical companies, health care organizations, and other qualifying groups. If you are interested in a custom book, including chapters from more than one of our titles, we can provide that service as well.

For details, please contact:
Special Sales Department, Springer Publishing Company, LLC
11 West 42nd Street, 15th Floor, New York, NY 10036-8002
Phone: 877-687-7476 or 212-431-4370; Fax: 212-941-7842
E-mail: sales@springerpub.com

Printed in the United States of America by Gasch Printing.

To triage nurses everywhere.

Few people can understand what you encounter each shift . . . the overwhelming and unpredictable influx of patients, the sights and sounds of distress, the stories that simply do not make sense . . . yet you professionally balance the chaos with flawless precision, making split-second decisions in the best interest of each patient. Your selfless acts, gentle hands, and compassionate hearts touch the lives of many. Your commitment to excellence is deserving of a book dedicated to you.

Contents

CONTENTS

Reviewers

Meredith Addison, MSN, RN,
    CEN, FAEN
Staff Nurse
Emergency Department
Regional Hospital
Terre Haute, Indiana

Jessica Castner, PhD, RN, CEN
Assistant Professor
University of Buffalo School
    of Nursing
Buffalo, New York

Mary Fardanesh, BSN, RN
Staff Nurse 1
Emergency Department
Kaiser Permanente South
    Sacramento Medical Center
Sacramento, California

Dawn Friedly Gray, MSN, RN,
    CEN, CCRN
Clinical Coordinator
Emergency Department
Paoli Hospital
Paoli, Pennsylvania

Dawn Hitchcock, MD
Board Certified in Emergency
    Medicine
California Emergency Physicians
Sutter Roseville Medical Center
Roseville, California

Deb Jeffries, MSN Ed, RN-BC,
    CEN, CPEN
Clinical Education Specialist
Banner Desert Medical Center
    Emergency Department
Cardon Children's Medical
    Center Emergency
    Department
Mesa, Arizona

Rebecca S. McNair, RN, CEN
President/Founder
Triage First, Inc.
Fairview, North Carolina

Michelle Michael-Korn, MS,
    RN, CEN
Director of Nursing
Emergency Services
Samaritan Medical Center
Watertown, New York

Wende M. Ryan, MS, RN-BC,
    CEN, CCRN
Clinical Educator, Critical Care
Rochester General Health
    Systems
Rochester, New York

REVIEWERS

Alexandra Schneider, PhD, PsyD, RN, FNP, LNCC, NY-SAFE
Honeoye Valley Family Practice
University of Rochester School of Nursing
Strong Memorial Hospital Emergency Room
Lima, New York

Nancy Shelton, BSN, RN, EMT-P
Emergency Department
St. Vincent's Hospital
Birmingham, Alabama

Andrew Wong, RN, CEN, CPEN
Staff Nurse
Lenox Hill Emergency Department
North Shore Long Island Jewish Health System
Woodside, New York

Foreword

In 2011, the American Nurses Association recognized emergency nursing as a specialty. Within that specialty, areas of focus have been developed to standardize the knowledge and practice base to enable a wide range of practitioners, from novice to expert, to provide excellent evidence-based clinical care across a wide spectrum of health care facilities—from small rural to large urban trauma centers. While standardization in some areas has been effected through courses such as the Trauma Nurse Core Course (TNCC), Emergency Nursing Pediatric Course (ENPC), and Advanced Cardiovascular Life Support (ACLS), the art and science of emergency nursing triage has had a longer period of development and standardization. Standardization in this field is critical because correct triage requires a broad knowledge base of *all* these areas, as well as excellent decision-making skills and tools.

Lynn Sayre Visser has devoted her career to emergency nursing, believing each patient deserves unbiased care that is nothing short of excellent. She has a "can-do, never give up, reach for the stars" mindset, which makes her an exemplary nursing role model. She has published in a variety of arenas, including emergency and radiology nursing, and she was a pilot reviewer for the American Association of Legal Nurse Consultants' learning modules.

Anna Sivo Montejano has a passion for health care delivered in the emergency setting. Her intense desire for quality triage, paired with her compelling enthusiasm for the teaching of others, has allowed her to touch lives across the emergency nursing continuum. She is making a difference: from delivering the highest quality patient care, to teaching students, to writing for publication.

Both Lynn Sayre Visser and Anna Sivo Montejano have shown purposeful and energetic devotion to the development of the art and science of emergency triage. Their enthusiasm and dedication to the holistic education of health care providers has my utmost admiration, and I consider them to be rising stars in this arena. Among the group of Triage First educators, they have consistently stood out as having the most excellent evaluations and have proven themselves worthy of a following.

Valerie Aarne Grossman, a published author in this field, has worked tirelessly since publishing her first edition of *Quick Reference to Triage* in 1998, with her second edition publishing in 2003. In 2005, she co-authored *Emergency Nursing: 5-Tier Triage Protocols,* with Julie K. Briggs. Both books have been translated into Japanese. She has served as a mentor to me and to others, not only in this area of focus, but also as a guide for those of us engaged in emergency nursing leadership and triage education. Ms. Grossman has worked behind the scenes in this way to further the art and science of triage, foregoing personal recognition in favor of promoting and educating others to join in this work.

These three author/editors join together in leading a line of nursing authors, researchers, and teachers of triage to present essential information for the triage nurse to access quickly and repeatedly. *Fast Facts for the Triage Nurse* covers every area of triage in a concise and professional manner, starting with the essentials of triage orientation, preceptorship, and self-care of the triage nurse, and including "Tips for Success at Triage," a chapter created using helpful snippets of triage information from national emergency nursing experts. The book goes on to address point-of-entry processes, nursing essentials, and current trends that impact the initial patient–nurse encounter and are useful in settings from urgent care to the emergency department. The final sections address "red flag" clinical presentations, special populations, and case studies to help the triage nurse understand these risky areas of triage nursing.

This book offers the opportunity to examine and discuss every aspect of triage nursing concepts and skills. "Fast Facts in a Nutshell" located throughout the book highlight critical information for easy reference. This book will be valuable for any nurse practicing triage.

Rebecca S. McNair, RN, CEN
President/Founder, Triage First, Inc.
Fairview, North Carolina

Preface

The purpose of this book is to provide new and seasoned nurses, preceptors, educators, and management teams with foundational skills that can be used throughout the triage orientation process as well as when practicing as an experienced triage nurse. Highlighted concepts include building confidence in the triage role, accurately assessing patient presentations, reducing personnel and hospital liability, increasing patient and staff satisfaction, and, ultimately, delivering quality patient care that supports best outcomes.

Triage is one of the toughest jobs in health care. Patients rarely present to triage with a diagnosis, but rather convey what is often a multitude of complaints, signs, and symptoms that must be weeded through to effectively determine how sick the patient really is. The authors of this book have years of experience practicing, teaching, and writing about triage to support the reader in the journey toward enhancing triage knowledge.

The main themes and objectives focus on numerous aspects of triage, from front-end processes and orientation to clinical practice and nursing essentials. The diverse factors of patient populations—age, gender, ethnicity, socioeconomic status, and so on—all impact the care a patient receives. A patient may present with a simple laceration, but a self-inflicted wound and a history of mental illness leads to safety issues for the patient and the individuals in his or her immediate environment. Patient care must be individualized to each patient for each visit. This book details the many aspects of triage in an organized manner using real-life examples to harden the facts.

The book is divided into parts to help organize the flow of information. The establishment of self-care and orientation early on sets the stage for a nurse to be successful in the triage setting. The sections cover workflow and "red flag" presentations, introduced in an organized manner with easy-to-find information. Each chapter contains a brief introduction as well as objectives, followed by "just the facts" information. Information that should not be missed is highlighted in "Fast Facts in a Nutshell" throughout the book. The term *provider* is threaded throughout the content and represents a medical doctor (MD), doctor of osteopathy (DO), nurse practitioner (NP), or physician assistant (PA). Treatment interventions are covered in various sections. However, each member of the health care team should only act within his or her scope of practice and follow facility protocols.

The authors, who have more than 80 years of combined nursing experience among them, share a common passion for the topic of triage. They reached out to other professionals around the country, who contributed and reviewed chapters, in their quest to bring this book to the highest possible level of functionality for the frontline triage nurse and others practicing triage. No other source is available on this topic that brings together the expertise of so many valuable professionals. Some readers may want to read this book cover to cover, while others may stick it in their lab coat pocket and pull it out for use as a quick resource to answer a clinical question. Perhaps it will be most helpful to novice readers, who will benefit from the concise expertise contained in this book before "learning it the hard way," one patient at a time.

Lynn Sayre Visser
Anna Sivo Montejano
Valerie Aarne Grossman

Acknowledgments

The authors collectively thank our editor, Elizabeth Nieginski, for embracing this project with energy, enthusiasm, and passion. Elizabeth, no words are remotely sufficient to express our gratitude for your diligent guidance, open arms, and willingness to consider each idea. We appreciate the entire Springer Publishing team for their meticulous efforts in creating the best possible product. To Rebecca and Michael McNair, for bringing this author team together: Your friendship and support means the world to us. To each contributor and reviewer for investing your expertise, time, and energy: Your detailed contribution to the content and your lightning-speed replies are much appreciated. We are grateful to the Emergency Nurses Association for the opportunities, knowledge, and growth each of us has experienced thanks to our affiliation with the organization. Lastly, we appreciate modern-day technology for regularly bringing together this East and West Coast team so we could create the vision, develop the manuscript, and fulfill the dream.

To this wonderful team of authors and dear friends: Each of us brought our unique gifts and individuality to the table, creating a joyful, stress-free experience. In early morning conference calls, from chit-chatting to getting down to business, we poured our hearts into producing a high-quality, informational triage book. This journey has been wild yet incredible . . . Dr. Search Engine, Ms. Analytical, and Ms. Eagle Eye . . . our talents blended seamlessly. What started as a simple idea has flourished into a book filled with knowledge and passion from caregivers around the country. We did it!

Lynn Sayre Visser: To the love of my life, my husband, Scott Visser, and to my children, Chase, Colton, and Brody: You light up my days with your laughter, creativity, and wonderful sense of humor. To my mom, dad, Cressey, and every patient, colleague, and mentor who has inspired me, challenged me, and changed me: I am humbly grateful for the gifts you have bestowed on me and for pushing me to fulfill my potential. To my dear friend, Jennifer Payan, for being the sister I always wanted; and to my family, extended family, and the other rocks in my life—you know who you are—no words will ever suffice to express my gratitude for your being by my side during life's ups and downs. I am eternally grateful.

Anna Sivo Montejano: First and most important, I would like to thank my wonderful husband, Phil, for supporting me throughout the past year with writing this book. You have made this journey a wonderful experience, thanks to your continued patience and understanding while I fulfilled this dream. To my amazing children, Zsuzsa, Michael, and Marcus: I am so fortunate to have three awesome kids like you. Yes, your mom is finally done with the book . . . time to celebrate! To Anyu, Apu, and family: Without any of you this would not have been possible. Thank you for your ongoing encouragement.

Valerie Aarne Grossman: No writer can devote her time to her desk and her project without the support from key people in her life. John and Marie Aarne: Thank you for your daily support and encouragement . . . there is no daughter who is more blessed than I am. Sarah Grossman, Nicole Grossman, and Jake Grant: Thank you for caring for our home while I have been sequestered at my desk for this past year . . . you kept life "normal" for me while I worked with my West Coast colleagues.

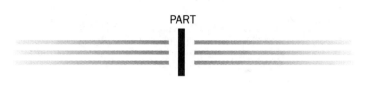

PART

I

Setting the Stage for Success at Triage

I

Orienting to Triage

Lynn Sayre Visser

Embarking on triage orientation is both an exciting and a scary time in a nurse's career, due to the geographical isolation of the triage area and the independent decision making required. Whether you practice in an emergency department (ED), urgent care center, telephone triage facility, or pre-hospital setting, new concepts intertwined with potentially different protocols and processes can leave you feeling uneasy. However, with a comprehensive orientation and the right perspective, the rewards that come with working in triage can be greater than the stressors imposed.

Since the triage nurse makes quick decisions that can be the difference between life and death, excellent critical thinking skills and judgment are essential. In addition, the triage nurse must have the ability to multitask while simultaneously considering the needs of patients, colleagues, and the department as a whole. Triage orientation is critical to high-quality patient outcomes and a nurse's success in the triage role.

Upon conclusion of this chapter, you will be able to:

1. Define triage
2. State the recommended qualifications for a triage nurse
3. State the purpose of triage orientation
4. Describe how to prepare for triage orientation
5. List resources available to enhance the triage education experience

WHAT IS TRIAGE?

Triage is a dynamic process. The word *triage* is derived from the French verb *trier*, which means "to sort." A person can be triaged anywhere, at any time, with only a moment's notice. A patient may be triaged in the ambulance bay, hospital parking lot, or on the floor of the waiting room. Triage is not isolated to one location but rather is a *process*; patients are sorted upon arrival and re-sorted frequently throughout their stay. Many practicing triage nurses find they informally triage patients all day long. This assessment takes place in the grocery store, health club, and while riding the elevator at work. Consider the person you see in the grocery store checkout line wearing flip flops. The pitting edema protruding beyond the flip flop straps is hard to miss. You begin to scan the person from head to toe. You focus on his or her respiratory effort and wonder what the pulse oximetry and heart rate might reveal. This practice of performing spontaneous assessments all day long develops as a habit for nurses and translates to valuable skills that can be utilized in the triage work setting. The goal of the triage nurse is to determine:

- How sick is the patient?
- How quickly does the patient need to be seen (determined by acuity level)?

Many health care facilities have a designated "triage room." This location is merely that—a room in which to store needed supplies that serves as a functional location for triage when the time is appropriate. However, the triage room must *never* be misinterpreted as the only place triage can occur. Triaging patients in the *most* appropriate setting and getting each patient to the right treatment location in the time frame necessary to promote best outcomes is a vital aspect of the triage nurse's role.

RECOMMENDED QUALIFICATIONS OF A TRIAGE NURSE

Before orienting to triage, the orientee and leadership or education team should determine if recommended qualifications to work in triage have been met. According to the Emergency Nurses Association (ENA; 2011), time as an ED nurse is not the determining factor for being qualified for triage; rather, experience in conjunction with formalized triage training, certifications, and specific qualities is recommended.

Qualifications

Recommended qualifications include (but are not limited to):

- Registered nurse
- Completion of a formalized triage training program
- Completion of a clinical orientation to triage with a dedicated preceptor

- Exceptional interpersonal, communication, and leadership skills
- Ability to multitask, collaborate, and work under stress
- Solid clinical and physical assessment skills
- Strong critical thinking and interviewing skills
- Ability to educate, delegate, and demonstrate sensitivity to cultural awareness
- For pediatric triage, an understanding of growth and development principles
- Understanding of facility policies and procedures, departmental flow, and treatment areas

Although ENA does not recommend a specific number of years of experience before orienting to triage, some triage education companies and facilities suggest a minimum of one year's experience at that specific facility before embarking on triage orientation.

COURSES AND CERTIFICATIONS

Courses and certifications that support the nurse in preparing for the triage role include:

- Certified emergency nurse (CEN)
- Certified pediatric emergency nurse (CPEN)
- Basic life support (BLS)
- Basic disaster life support (BDLS)
- Advanced cardiac life support (ACLS)
- Advanced disaster life support (ADLS)
- Emergency nurse pediatric course (ENPC)
- Pediatric advanced life support (PALS)
- Geriatric emergency nurse education (GENE)
- Trauma nurse core course (TNCC)
- Other courses mandated by your organization or governing agencies

FAST FACTS in a NUTSHELL

Active membership in at least one professional nursing organization (e.g., Emergency Nurses Association) creates a strong foundation for continued growth within the nursing profession. Networking opportunities, listserv access, and educational offerings will help you develop into the triage nurse you want to be!

PURPOSE OF TRIAGE ORIENTATION

A thorough orientation to triage provides the foundational skills upon which to build in the months and years ahead. The orientation should be designed to prepare a person for success and serves many purposes that include:

Understanding the Triage Role

- Gaining confidence in the triage role
- Decreasing stress by developing an understanding of the triage nurse role
- Acquiring tips for enhancing productivity at triage
- Improving job satisfaction

Advancing Current Knowledge

- Developing strong customer service techniques to utilize at triage
- Gaining awareness about compassion fatigue and empathy burnout
- Managing families and their reactions to stress
- Understanding how cultural beliefs and language barriers impact the delivery of care
- Developing competency and improving patient care outcomes
- Learning how to initiate advanced triage protocols

Understanding Triage Flow

- Prioritizing an influx of patients in a short time frame
- Learning when to perform a rapid triage assessment versus a comprehensive triage assessment
- Understanding patient flow, acuity assignment, and priority setting
- Learning how to work with a physician, physician assistant, or nurse practitioner at triage

Identifying "Red Flag" Patient Presentations and Enhancing Documentation Skills

- Gaining awareness of high-acuity presentations and concerning red flag findings
- Learning how to best document chief complaints and associated symptoms
- Acquiring tips on working with the electronic medical record (EMR)
- Developing skills to keep patients and staff safe

Understanding Policies and Procedures

- Understanding legal concerns (e.g., provisions of the Emergency Medical Treatment and Active Labor Act [EMTALA]) in order to decrease liability
- Gaining knowledge in the medical screening exam (MSE)
- Understanding facility policies, procedures, and resource availability
  - Availability of a labor and delivery department, cardiac catheterization lab, trauma team, and so on

TRIAGE ORIENTATION

In preparing for triage orientation, the orientee may or may not have an opportunity to choose who shows him or her the ins and outs of triage. Nursing leadership or educators should be actively involved in carefully selecting triage preceptors. The preceptors chosen should be role model staff members who are passionate about teaching and who meet the recommended triage qualifications. From the time we are children, our parents, teachers, coaches, friends, and family share their wisdom, shaping us into the individuals we become. Nursing is the same in that our practice is strongly influenced by other nursing professionals. The right preceptor can make all the difference in a person's orientation and future success at triage.

=====*FAST FACTS in a NUTSHELL*

- Advanced planning to prepare for triage orientation and ensuring a good preceptor–orientee match is paramount.
- Triage orientation should involve preceptors who will guide, challenge, and support the learning process. Gaining knowledge and exposure to a multitude of experiences during the triage orientation best prepares a person for success at triage.

Selecting the Right Preceptors for Triage Orientation

Triage is an art that requires continued growth and development. When contemplating which staff might be best for orienting nurses to triage, consider the following:

- Does the person have sufficient triage experience?
- Is the person enthusiastic and does he or she have the desire to precept with a positive attitude?

- Does the preceptor meet the recommended triage qualifications?
- Does the person possess effective communication skills?
- Is the person respected by peers for his or her priority-setting abilities at triage?
- Can you envision this person giving constructive criticism?
- Does the person possess excellent clinical and critical thinking skills?
- Is the person open to receiving constructive criticism?
- Is the person knowledgeable about ED flow?
- Will the person push the orientee to his or her potential?
- Does the person consistently identify unstable patients and assign appropriate acuity levels?
- Is the person self-motivated to learn and advance his or her precepting and nursing skills?
- Has the person attended preceptor courses and gained knowledge in adult learning principles?
- Will the preceptor maximize the orientation time?

Difficulties can arise between the preceptor and orientee during triage orientation when differences exist, including:

- Expectations
- Values and beliefs
- Personalities
- Past life experiences
- Cultural backgrounds
- Generational differences
- Variation in learning and teaching styles

Efforts to create a positive learning experience for the orientee should be made. Being aware of these differences can help management teams and nurse-educators best match the preceptor and orientee.

Communication

Communication *throughout* the triage orientation is essential. Although your organization may have clear objectives for orientation, the orientee should develop personal objectives that are communicated to the preceptor. If the orientee's goals are clearly expressed, the preceptor can best help the orientee achieve them. At times during the orientation, miscommunication may occur. Building the relationship on open, honest communication is imperative. A manager or nurse educator should follow up with the orientee and preceptor to provide support and evaluate if the orientation is meeting the expectations of all involved.

Equipment Lists

Knowing where to find supplies and emergency equipment in the triage area is critical. The unique layout of the triage area often creates systems that may not be uniform with other supplies within the facility. Ensure familiarity with the location of basic equipment, including the following:

- Emergency supplies such as oral airways, bag valve mask, crash cart, and delivery tray
- Code blue button, panic button, emergency numbers
- Hard cervical collars and backboards
- Electrocardiogram machine
- Blood pressure cuffs and pulse oximeters in all sizes
- Blood glucose machines
- Emesis basins, specimen cups, bandaging supplies (e.g., gauze, scissors, saline, etc.)
- Personal protective equipment (e.g., gloves, gowns, face shields, etc.)
- Downtime slips and paperwork in case of EMR updates or system failure

Teamwork

Although triage may be a geographically isolated area, the role the triage nurse plays is an integral component of the treatment team. Communication with the charge nurse or patient flow coordinator regarding incoming patients and their acuity levels is critical to departmental flow and patient safety. A successful triage orientation requires a team approach to ensure the orientee grasps essential concepts and understands processes unique to the triage area. Acquiring the skills needed to effectively function at triage is beneficial to other staff on the treatment team once the orientee is practicing solo. Thus, throughout this book, content covered will build critical thinking skills and cover key concepts to support success at triage.

COMPLETION OF TRIAGE ORIENTATION

Completion of the triage orientation is the first step in beginning a new chapter of nursing experiences. The challenges posed at triage are unlike any others. Often, the triage nurse is the first clinical person who sets the tone for the patient experience and patient outcome. Working with the human dynamics of patients and families in a time of crisis can be overwhelming, but the triage nurse has a unique opportunity to make a difference in the lives of others. Providing each patient presenting to triage with an accurate, unbiased, and nonjudgmental assessment, coupled with caring and compassion, is vital to every patient encounter.

Remember, even though orientation may be complete, the learning should never stop. As time allows, seek the opportunity to perform real-time follow-up on patient presentations or conduct retrospective chart reviews to learn from your triage assessments and acuity level assignments. Comparing your triage decision making with the patient's final diagnoses will provide invaluable insight that can help with future triage. Even the most seasoned and experienced triage nurses have times of uncertainty in the triage role. No nurse is ever too old, too smart, or too experienced to consult with a fellow nurse or medical provider. A commitment to lifelong learning is imperative to your role in nursing and is a critical component to growing into an exceptional triage nurse.

FAST FACTS in a NUTSHELL

- Each patient presenting for medical care deserves an unbiased assessment.
- Personal judgments should not influence triage decision making.
- Although the triage assignment may feel isolating at times, the triage nurse is an integral part of the team.
- Always strive to keep learning and better your patient assessment skills.

RESOURCES

Although your facility may have a triage orientation program, additional resources to support triage education can be valuable. The "Resources" section at the end of this text offers other ideas for enhancing the orientation. These resources include formalized live or online triage education programs, books, and websites.

REFERENCE

Emergency Nurses Association. (2011). Triage qualifications position statement. Retrieved May 9, 2014, from www.ena.org

2

Precepting at Triage

Lynn Sayre Visser

Precepting an individual at triage is an opportunity to shape that nurse's future practice. When the orientee begins practicing on his or her own in triage, this nurse may make potentially life-threatening or life-altering decisions about your family members and friends. Therefore, giving the orientee the experiences and education that you would want every nurse to have at triage is crucial. This chapter covers essential skills required of the preceptor and provides tips for creating a positive experience for the triage orientee.

Upon conclusion of this chapter, you will be able to:

1. Explain adult teaching principles
2. Understand the impact of generational differences in the workplace
3. List recommended qualifications for a triage preceptor
4. Explain benefits of precepting at triage
5. Describe components of the triage orientation

ADULT TEACHING AND LEARNING PRINCIPLES

Recognizing that adults do not all acquire new knowledge in a similar manner is fundamental to becoming an excellent preceptor. Individuals come to learning situations with varying past experiences and knowledge upon which to build. Understanding the foundation of work and life experience that the individual possesses is important.

Learning Styles

Learning styles vary among individuals. "Learning style refers to the unique way in which a person perceives, interacts with, and responds to a learning situation" (Billings & Halstead, 2009, p. 23). Some adults may know how they learn best while others may be lacking that insight. As a preceptor, being aware of the unique needs of an individual is vital to laying the groundwork for a caring, mutually respectful relationship. Understanding students personally and professionally, their interests, and how they will best engage in the learning experience helps the preceptor work with each individual.

Adult learning theory supports frequent use of a combination of these learning styles:

- Visual
- Auditory
- Kinesthetic (hands-on application)

Fortunately, triage orientation provides an opportunity to regularly incorporate all three of these learning needs. However, knowledge of the orientee's learning style will help the preceptor seek opportunities to meet the individual's needs. Getting orientees involved in the learning process is critical to their success; thus, the more orientation can be fine-tuned to meet individual needs, the more engaged the person will likely be.

Important principles of adult learning include:

- Positive reinforcement
- Recognition that adults learn at different speeds (Thoms, 2012)

Asking the Right Questions

Asking the orientee to share the learning methods that are most effective for him or her and the expectations the orientee has for the orientation sets the tone for a positive orientee–preceptor relationship. This approach opens the lines of communication between the orientee and preceptor. Questions to ask the orientee *throughout* the orientation include:

- What are your goals for the triage orientation?
- Is auditory or visual learning better for you or do you prefer both?
- Is the hands-on aspect of learning crucial to your success?
- What can I do as a preceptor to ensure I meet your learning needs?
- Do you have any barriers to learning that I should be aware of?
- Do you have previous experience in triage?
- What is a worry you have about working in triage?
- Do you have fears or misconceptions I can try to alleviate?
- What do you like to do in your spare time?

Although inquiring about interests outside the workplace may seem irrelevant, this question opens the door for finding common interests with the orientee and demonstrates your investment in the person as a whole. Outside interests also serve as an outlet for stress release, which is crucial for any individual. Additionally, the preceptor may learn about other relevant life experiences (e.g., work as a paramedic, customer service representative, sales manager) that may influence the individual's performance in the triage role.

Supporting the Orientee

Patience as a preceptor is essential. We all started with limited triage knowledge. Each triage took longer as a new triage nurse. We may have failed to ask the right questions. Maybe a patient was undertriaged or overtriaged or the essential clinical assessment was missed. Gaining knowledge from each experience is part of the learning process. During orientation, providing the orientee with the same level of support you received or wished you had received while on triage orientation will help foster confidence in and prepare the new orientee to practice on his or her own. Provide positive reinforcement and constructive feedback when appropriate and maintain an awareness of both verbal and nonverbal communication. Sharing your expertise is a gift that does not stop. The knowledge you impart to others will potentially be shared and continue to influence the practice of nurses over time.

==========*FAST FACTS in a NUTSHELL*

Be patient with individuals who are orienting to triage. Let the orientee see your passion for triage and enthusiasm for sharing knowledge with others.

THE GENERATIONAL DIVIDE

The profession of nursing is currently influenced by nurses from four generations. Veterans, baby boomers, generation X, and generation Y nurses work side by side yet reflect different upbringings, belief systems, and values. Generational differences can create challenges in the workplace if these variances are not recognized. Thus, understanding the differences and similarities between the generations and how to instill a cohesive team environment will help preceptors perform. Table 2.1 illustrates these important generational variations.

Increasing utilization of technology in health care can certainly create challenges for nurse educators and preceptors. Varying comfort levels with technology and adaptations to technology training sessions will most likely need to be made. For example, if an

TABLE 2.1 The Four Generations in Nursing

Generation	Year Born	Colloquial Name	Life Experiences	Characteristics	Approach to New Technology
Veterans	1925–1945	"Silent Generation"	Experienced World War II and the Great Depression in childhood	Hard working Disciplined Dedicated	Slow to learn new technology
Baby boomers	1946–1964		Came of age during civil rights protests Caring for kids and aging parents	Question authority Risk takers Feel fulfilled through work	Slow to learn new technology
Generation X	1965–1980		Many were raised in single-parent families that were money conscious Exposed to technology in their teen years	Independent Self-reliant Self-motivated Instant gratification Desire mentoring Enjoy work/life balance	Understand technology but are slower to adapt than their generation Y counterparts
Generation Y	1981–2000	"Net Generation" "Millennials"	Grew up with technology	Multitaskers Desire for constant feedback Enjoy work/life balance	Adapt to new technology easily Expect others to use technology

electronic medical record (EMR) is utilized at your facility, the orientee may require one-on-one interaction or additional time learning the computer system.

RECOMMENDED QUALIFICATIONS FOR A TRIAGE PRECEPTOR

Precepting at triage should be a role that is fulfilled by well-qualified individuals who possess a "can-do" attitude. A person's years of experience at triage should not be the deciding factor in determining whether he or she is capable of precepting but rather clinical expertise coupled with enthusiasm and a passion for teaching. Knowledge is gained most easily when energy and excitement for the topic is conveyed (Svinicki & McKeachie, 2011). Recommended qualifications for the triage preceptor are discussed in Chapter 1.

Desired Traits in a Triage Preceptor

Additional traits of a triage preceptor include:

- Reliability
- Clinical excellence
- Approachability
- Compassion and empathy
- Enthusiasm
- Familiarity with generational differences
- Clinical excellence
- Strong communication/customer service skills
- Self-motivation

BENEFITS OF PRECEPTING

Staff who precept orientees experience many benefits. Some of the rewards noted may include:

- Personal satisfaction from helping the orientee develop professionally
- Opportunity to share knowledge with other nurses
- Growth of self-knowledge derived from the need to understand and explain triage concepts
- Further development of critical thinking skills
- Recognition from peers and managers
- Career advancement
- Financial incentives

IDEAS FOR THE ORIENTATION

By the time the orientee is ready for the didactic portion of the triage clinical orientation, it is to be hoped that some classroom training has been completed and the orientee has a general understanding of triage policies and procedures, acuity level assignment, and the unique aspects of the triage area. During the orientation process, the preceptor should maximize the time spent with the orientee. Ways to effectively use the orientation time include learning about available resources, policies and procedures, and skills and processes.

Resources

- Have the orientee:
  - Go on a scavenger hunt to find needed triage supplies
  - Locate electrocardiogram machines and wheelchairs
  - Learn where supplies needed to stock the triage area are located
- Discuss with the orientee:
  - The availability of security (e.g., panic buttons, emergency numbers)
  - Use of notification devices (e.g., code blue button, walkie-talkies)
  - Continuing education opportunities and how to access them

Policies and Procedures

- Explain legal concerns at triage, including the Emergency Medical Treatment and Active Labor Act (EMTALA) and the medical screening exam
- Discuss mandated documentation for triage
- Review requirements for paperwork and the EMR
- Review triage acuity level policies and procedures
- Evaluate the orientee's understanding of triage acuity levels
- Review policies for common patient circumstances (e.g., "left without being seen," "against medical advice," etc.)
- Review the facility's advanced triage protocols
- Discuss facility-specific limitations (e.g., no labor and delivery capability, no trauma surgeon availability, etc.)
- Review disaster policies and resources
- Discuss facility lockdown policy and procedures

Skills and Processes

- Discuss and role model the triage process and patient flow
- Discuss how to work with other staff at triage (e.g., providers, unlicensed personnel, etc.)

- Review the importance of communication and active listening at triage
- Discuss trauma at triage, team members to activate, who to call, and patient placement
- Review "red flag" patient presentations and questions and assessments to consider
- Discuss and demonstrate the use of customer service skills at triage
- Demonstrate differences when triaging adult, pediatric, and geriatric patients
- Observe the orientee during triage of adult, pediatric, and geriatric patients
- Review self-care practices (e.g., stress alleviation, avoiding burnout, and compassion fatigue)

Evaluation Techniques

- Discuss the value of self-reflection to enhance the learning experience
- Discuss tools for orientee evaluation
- Perform chart reviews and evaluate the appropriateness of the triage acuity level assigned

Additional examples of points to consider during the triage orientation will be threaded throughout future chapters and can help in developing the orientation.

COMPLETION OF TRIAGE ORIENTATION

During the triage orientation, evaluation tools should be utilized to aid in determining if the orientee is ready for the triage assignment. As a preceptor, your responsibility is to ensure that the orientee is only signed off for triage once orientation objectives are met. These objectives will vary by facility. Although formal written tools will likely be utilized in the evaluation process, informal conversations throughout the triage orientation are also important. Consider the tips below for effectively communicating with orientees.

Crucial Conversations

Crucial conversations regarding the orientee's performance can be challenging. However, accurately evaluating the orientee for safe practice at triage is an essential component of precepting. When speaking to an orientee who is having difficulty, use the following guidelines:

- *Provide timely feedback:* Regular, constructive feedback will minimize surprises at the end of the orientation. Set orientees up to succeed . . . and if all else fails, let them know where they stand on a *regular* basis. No one wants to feel they were blind-sided at the end of an orientation period, and this practice will alleviate stress for both the preceptor and orientee.

- *Control emotions and avoid defensive behavior:* Mastering this skill can be challenging, especially when experiencing frustration with an orientee. The preceptor needs to think about what to say and how to say it before approaching the orientee. Put yourself in the position of the orientee and think about how the information will be perceived.
- *Address the right problem:* Consider what needs to be tackled so the right results can be achieved.
- *Change the orientee's perspective:* If the orientee's performance raises concerns about patient safety, consider explaining how his or her behavior can potentially impact the patient outcome. The preceptor should think, "What are the consequences of the behavior?" and address the concerns with the orientee.

Giving Praise

Praise is also a critical element of the orientation. Even an orientee who excels will want to know where he or she stands. Some may think no news is good news, but is that enough? Praise serves as both a reward and a motivational tool and should be delivered appropriately to have the greatest impact.

- *Prepare to give praise:* This meaningful moment should receive the same or more preparation as delivering constructive criticism. Make your comments count!
- *Be specific:* Set your standards and expectations early in the orientation and compliment the orientee when expectations are being met. For example, explain that *when* you triaged the patient, *what happened* was you picked up on the subtle symptoms raising concern of a myocardial infarction, and *the result of your actions* was the identification of a potentially life-threatening condition. When you add that the patient went into cardiac arrest the minute he or she was placed on the ED gurney, your orientee will feel his or her actions in identifying the sick patient were appropriate!
- *Timely feedback:* Timeliness is essential in providing praise so the orientee remembers the details of the situation. Praise also gives momentum for continuing to perform well and builds confidence.

TIPS FOR NURSING LEADERSHIP AND NURSING EDUCATORS

Ways to support your preceptors include:

- Providing preceptors with training in adult teaching and learning principles, effective communication skills, and conflict management
- Dedicating time to the review of standards of care and policies and procedures
- Selecting preceptors who meet facility or nationally recommended triage qualifications
- Listening to the preceptor if concerns about the orientee arise
- Checking in with the preceptor throughout the orientation so no surprises develop regarding the orientee's performance
- Considering generational, cultural, and personality differences before matching preceptors and orientees
- Having a pool of triage preceptors from which to select to avoid preceptor burnout
- Providing preceptor training in how best to utilize department resources
- Developing a preceptor committee to enhance communication and ensure the same orientation principles are implemented by all preceptors (e.g., feedback, praise, etc.)

=====*FAST FACTS in a NUTSHELL*

- As a preceptor, commit to being a lifelong learner. To keep up with the ever-changing health care system you must seek learning opportunities and attend continuing education courses.
- Orientees often say knowledge is gained most easily when energy and excitement is relayed by the preceptor. Be a role model!
- Empathize with the orientee. Provide the level of high quality training that you would want for yourself.

REFERENCE

Billings, D. M., & Halstead, J. A. (2009). *Teaching in nursing: A guide for faculty.* (3rd ed.). St Louis, MO: Elsevier Saunders.

Svinicki, M., & McKeachie, W. J. (2011). *McKeachie's teaching tips: Strategies, research, and theory for college and university teachers* (13th ed.). Belmont, CA: Wadsworth.

Thoms, K. They're not just big kids: Motivating adult learners. Retrieved March 18, 2012, from http://frank.mtsu.edu/~itconf/.htmlroceed/01/22

Weingarten, R. M. & Weingarten, C. T. (2013). Generational diversity in ED and education settings: A daughter–mother perspective. *Journal of Emergency Nursing, 39*(4), 369–371.

3

Tips for Success at Triage

Lynn Sayre Visser and Anna Sivo Montejano

Working in triage can be overwhelming. The fast-paced environment, vast knowledge required, and the unpredictable nature of the triage area can leave even seasoned triage nurses feeling the stress. Emergency nursing leaders were asked to share their techniques for delivering quality care at triage, how they nurture themselves while in the triage role, and how they promote efficient departmental flow, all while keeping patient safety as the primary goal. This chapter includes tips, wisdom, and insight from nurses who have worked in the trenches and their suggestions for setting oneself up for success at triage.

Upon conclusion of this chapter, you will be able to:

1. Identify a minimum of three tips you can incorporate into your triage practice
2. Reflect on your own triage success tips that you can share with other triage nurses
3. Identify one method of sharing triage tips that can be incorporated in your facility

TRIAGE TIPS AND RATIONALE

Rebecca S. McNair, RN, CEN, Fairview, North Carolina

- Obtain as much clinical education as possible, including advanced cardiac life support training, trauma nurse core course, emergency nurse pediatric course, and especially your certified emergency nurse (CEN) certification. The more clinical knowledge you have, the better prepared you will be to accurately and confidently triage any presentation.
- Engage in professional organizations for professional nursing development. Triage and any point-of-entry process requires a holistic and well-developed framework to be highly successful.

- Complete a formal, standardized triage course. A conceptual grasp of the knowledge and skills necessary ensures accurate triage acuity level assignment and disposition.

Polly Gerber Zimmermann, MS, MBA, RN, CEN, FAEN, Chicago, Illinois

- When building rapport with pediatric patients, you can't go wrong overestimating a young child's age. "Are you 7? Oh, only 5. Well, you seem like such a big boy!" You also can't go wrong telling parents what a cute and nice baby they have. What to do if the baby is not "pretty"? Say, "That is *some* baby" or compliment the cute outfit. Now you've started on the right foot, by showing how perceptive and smart you are as a nurse!
- Insist on a lunch break. I routinely worked 12-hour shifts without any break when things were hectic, to avoid the perception that the triage nurse was "sitting" while the rest of staff were "running around." Keep drinking water throughout the shift regardless. One of the first signs of dehydration is fatigue. Everyone needs a break. Even 5 minutes away will make you more effective.
- Toward the end of the triage interaction use a scripted phrase to show you care. My favorites are "That looks sore"; "I'm sorry this happened to you. I'm sure you didn't plan to be here"; or, "We'll take good care of you." This approach works to reassure the patient and show your empathy without trying to be original and creative when you are busy.
- Overestimate the time for anything (obtaining a bed, seeing the physician, going to radiology, etc.). Patients respond more positively when something happens before they expect it. No one likes to be the bearer of unpleasant news, so the temptation is strong to underestimate the time it will take for actions to occur. In the end, though, this just irritates patients more.
- The seriously ill are sometimes too sick to speak up. Therefore, do what you are supposed to do, whether you think it is needed or not. By checking all newly arrived patients, I found a patient who had been transported by ambulance with "hysterical back pain" who had rapidly progressing Guillain-Barré syndrome. By always doing an across-the-room assessment, I discovered a dusky infant with bradycardia and an asthmatic patient just before respiratory arrest occurred. The consistent theme was that none of them were asking for help.

Ensure the triage nurse receives regular breaks. When a person feels run down, critical thinking skills may be impaired and compassion and caring can be difficult to deliver. Breaks recharge an individual so high-quality patient care can be provided.

Reneé Semonin Holleran, PhD, FNP-BC, CEN, CCRN (alumnus), CFRN and CTRN (retired), FAEN, Former Editor-in-Chief, Journal of Emergency Nursing (2006–2013), Salt Lake City, Utah

- Listen to what patients tell you about their problems. Take a brief history to go along with the chief complaint. PQRST is a great tool for this. Most of the time the patient will tell you what is wrong. The physical assessment or other tests only confirm it.
- Today patients are on a plethora of medications prescribed by multiple providers. These medications are mixed in with over-the-counter medications that cause serious and often chronic side effects that frequently are worked up over and over again. Medications and medication interactions cause many problems that are often mistaken for something else.
- Caring and compassion can go a long way in getting you through a long shift. It takes more effort to be rude than to be kind.

Shelley Cohen, MSN, RN, CEN, Hohenwald, Tennessee

- Never make an assumption based on only one sense (what you see, hear, smell, touch). What looks, sounds, smells, and feels normal in and of itself may actually be a "red flag" finding when you engage *all* of your senses.
- Never hesitate to collaborate with a peer or provider on duty when unsure of a triage decision. The triage nurse cannot operate in a vacuum (isolation). Although physically the triage nurse typically works independently of other team members, always reach out for another opinion when needed.
- Learn to document your triage note in a manner that validates your triage decision. The only person who can clinically capture the patient presentation at the time of triage is the triage nurse. When retrospective review is required for legal or other purposes, you want to be sure your words "paint a picture" of this patient's status at the time of triage.

Dawn Friedly Gray, MSN, RN, CEN, CCRN, Paoli, Pennsylvania

- Find a way to show compassion and caring to every patient you triage. Triage is the first and the most important interaction in setting the tone for your patient's visit. Making a connection, valuing, and attempting to see why a patient is there through his or her eyes builds trust in the patient–nurse relationship.
- Trust your gut. Sometimes there is no specific clinical presentation or answer to a question that can "explain" why you feel someone needs immediate attention. Following your nursing instincts can save a life. Better to follow one's gut than to regret the decision later.
- You can learn something new every time you triage. Be open to learning and take the time to follow up to see if your assessment was appropriate. We should never stop learning and growing as nurses. Taking the time to review and reflect on our clinical decision making makes us stronger and keeps us attuned to our own "humanness." It helps us avoid judgmental attitudes and promotes ongoing professional development.

Deb Jeffries, MSN Ed, RN-BC, CEN, CPEN, Mesa, Arizona

- Keep an open mind; the "been there, done that, I've seen this a million times before" attitude will end up burning you. It is inherent in what nurses do that we categorize patients by chief complaint, symptom clusters, and the appropriate corresponding objective assessment. However, we must always be on guard to avoid categorizing and prioritizing patients based on invalid factors such as "drug seekers," "people who are overreacting," and "attention seekers."
- Delete the word "just" from your vocabulary and your thinking when you are at triage. If I could influence one last thing in my career it would be to eradicate the word "just" from the mindset of every triage nurse worldwide. The word "just" influences, albeit subtly sometimes, how we look at, assess, and determine prioritization of care for the patient. Phrases like "he's just drunk" and "he's just a drug seeker" will affect how we think about the patient. At triage there is *no one* who is "just" anything.
- Use a systematic approach to everything you do at triage. Using a consistent, systematic approach will help ensure that you do not miss anything. Whether it is how you obtain subjective and objective assessments or how you facilitate reassessments on patients awaiting treatment area placement, a systematic approach will help you go home at the end of your shift knowing that you have provided the best care possible to all those you have triaged.

Valerie Aarne Grossman, BSN, RN, MALS, NE-BC, Rochester, New York

- Never act surprised by anything you hear, see, smell, or touch. By maintaining professionalism at all times, you encourage the patient and family to trust that you are sensitive to their situation, and building a rapport with them will occur more easily.
- Remember that you are always on stage. You may be the first professional that patients and families see when they enter the hospital, and you may set the tone for their entire stay. If they see that you are a professional, and treat all others with respect, they will be more open to answering your questions honestly and facilitating your ability to triage effectively.
- Hear what the patients are saying; they live with their bodies and their lives more than you do. Not everything we hear in triage makes sense to us. However, don't assume that you are smarter than the patient when it comes to his or her body or life. If the patient says something that doesn't make sense, ask a few more questions instead of being quick to pass judgment on him or her.

Anna Sivo Montejano, MSN Ed, RN, CEN, El Dorado Hills, California

- Whenever a patient is placed in the triage room, make sure the patient enters first and then the nurse follows. If the nurse needs to exit quickly, due to a dangerous situation, it is easier to do so without the patient blocking the exit. Consider this when escorting a patient to an emergency department or urgent care bed. Always think "Safety First." Some patients may be unpredictable, leaving you trapped in the room with no way out!
- No matter what a patient tells you, never appear shocked. This may make the patient feel very uncomfortable. Have the attitude, "I see or hear this all the time!" It can be difficult for a patient to seek help, especially in an embarrassing situation.
- Always put on your "happy face" when greeting your triage patients. Patients may be going through a very stressful situation. They need someone who is compassionate and caring, not a cranky, irritable nurse who presents himself or herself as rude and unkind.
- Overexaggerate when asking patients if they drink alcohol. It's easier for a patient to admit to drinking less than more. Asking whether a patient normally drinks 2 liters of whisky a day leaves the patient feeling better, as he or she can reply, "Oh no, just one liter." He or she will also be more honest.
- When evaluating the use of drugs, maintain a matter-of-fact expression, as if you were questioning a person about shortness of

breath or chest pain. It is easier for the patient to answer without the addition of a nonverbal stigma being applied. Expressing to the patient, both verbally and nonverbally, that this is "simply a fact" may make it easier for a patient to admit to a drug history.

Lynn Sayre Visser, MSN, BS, RN, CEN, CPEN, CLNC, Loomis, California

- Triage is too complex to take the "see one, do one, teach one" approach to orientation. Attending a formalized triage education course should be the foundation of a person's triage orientation and can benefit seasoned triage nurses, too! Once the principles of triage are understood, the appropriate application of concepts in the clinical setting can best be achieved.
- When "the bus lets off" and the waiting room is packed wall to wall, often the tension builds among the triage team. When every second counts more than ever, one must never forget to see each arriving patient as an individual. A compassionate touch of a hand, a warm smile, or a genuine look of concern can go miles toward earning the respect of those waiting. Building rapport with the waiting room crowd is essential to survival at triage! When you set the right tone with each person upon arrival, those in the waiting room will "have your back" if a belligerent patient or irate customer steps your way.
- Some of the most treasured gifts I have received in my career have come from my work at triage. No words can adequately represent the personal satisfaction that comes with *recognizing* the person with an atypical myocardial infarction, the fetus in danger, or the subtle clues of intimate partner violence and then *acting* in the best interest of the patient. Cherishing the moments where you make a difference in the patient's outcome will help carry you through the tougher triage shifts.
- Invest in good quality shoes. Find a triage mentor. Share cases. Reflect on your triage shifts. Learn from mistakes. Never think you are too seasoned to mess up. We all have times when we fall flat on our faces. It's the journey—both triumphs and failures—that ultimately make us the best triage nurses we can be.

REFLECTION

Reflection is an essential component of professional growth. Learning from past experiences provides opportunity to incorporate knowledge gained into future practice. This chapter encompasses triage tips from nurses who have worked in the trenches and have learned through their experiences how to succeed during a shift in triage.

What triage tips do you have that you can bestow on others? We challenge you to reflect on your own practice and share triage tips with co-workers at your facility.

- Develop a bulletin board where staff can post their ideas.
- Share a tip of the day at change of shift.
- Create a "Triage Tip Binder" that all triage staff can access in the triage area.

As we each reflect on what has and has not worked for us at triage, we can create a better, safer, higher quality triage area and change the face of triage . . . one tip at a time!

FAST FACTS in a NUTSHELL

- Compassion and caring should be hallmarks of the care you deliver.
- Ongoing reflection is the key to fine-tuning your triage practice.
- If a patient presentation seems perplexing, consult with a colleague or medical provider. You should never feel alone at triage, but rather should seek the help you need to act in the best interest of the patient . . . *always*.

Personal Awareness for the Triage Nurse

Anna Sivo Montejano

Working in a stressful environment like triage can take a toll on a person. Self-awareness of one's emotions, feelings, and behavior is vital if the triage nurse is to function effectively. Irrespective of whether a nurse works in an urgent care center, an emergency department, or as a telephone triage nurse, stressors impact individuals differently. The effects of these stressors can appear insignificant initially, but the overwhelming emotions the nurse experiences daily can lead to physical or psychological crisis. Being aware of these factors can assist the nurse in keeping balance in his or her life.

Upon conclusion of this chapter, you will be able to:

1. Define compassion fatigue
2. Describe examples of how lateral violence affects patients
3. Explain empathy burnout

COMPASSION FATIGUE

Health care providers are confronted daily with emotionally challenging situations, which can tear at one's inner soul. We hear stories of pain, loss, and fear while often simultaneously seeing the tears of our patients and their families. Containing our own emotions can be difficult at times. How do health care providers suppress the anguish that is a part of their daily routine? Recognizing that health care providers are at risk for compassion fatigue is important.

Compassion fatigue results from caring for individuals with physical and emotional suffering, which diminishes the care providers' emotional, physical, and spiritual well-being.

Populations Vulnerable to Compassion Fatigue

- Police officers
- Emergency department personnel
- Firefighters
- Intensive care personnel
- Chaplains
- First responders

Signs and Symptoms of Compassion Fatigue

- Easily frustrated or irritated
- Physical, emotional, and mental exhaustion
- Difficulty getting to work
- Diminished interaction with others
- Losing compassion
- Feeling tired even after a good sleep

Prevention of Compassion Fatigue

Understanding the intricacies of compassion fatigue can help health care providers cope with their emotions rather than concealing them. A path of self-destruction can develop if the symptoms are not addressed appropriately. The treatment for compassion fatigue includes:

- Exercise
- Articulating your needs
- Adequate sleep
- Taking care of yourself
- Seeking support from others
- Validating your feelings with others who can relate
- Obtaining medical help if needed, but *do not self-medicate*

FAST FACTS in a NUTSHELL

- Awareness of physical and emotional pain experienced can lead to identifying compassion fatigue.
- Early identification of compassion fatigue signs and symptoms can lead to appropriate intervention and a return to a healthy lifestyle.

Lateral violence, also termed "horizontal violence," is bullying in the workplace. Lateral violence can cause stress and intimidation toward the victim. If experienced on a continuous basis, lateral violence may cause individuals to leave the profession of nursing.

Three Forms of Lateral Violence

- Physical
  - Inappropriate sexual innuendoes and touching (e.g., unwanted back rubbing)
- Verbal
  - Condescending comments
  - Verbal attacks
  - Rude comments
- Psychological
  - Attacks on one's integrity
  - Refusing to offer assistance
  - Eye rolling
  - Not working as a team
  - Gossiping about the individual
  - Being judged constantly

You may have experienced one or more forms of lateral violence at some point in your career. Perhaps you assigned a high acuity level to a patient and were met with derogatory comments from co-workers. As professionals, we must remember that often the entire picture is not visible to the eye. For example, consider a patient who arrives with minimal swelling to the forearm following an insect bite. One nurse may be quick to judge that this should be a low acuity patient. But when the patient's high blood pressure and additional symptoms— including a headache—are considered, the need for a higher acuity level becomes apparent. Comments from other staff regarding triage decision making should be withheld unless a patient is endangered or criticism is constructive.

Possible Consequences of Lateral Violence

- Errors (e.g., medication, lack of interventions)
- High rate of absenteeism
- Increased staff turnover
- Decreased job satisfaction
- Inadequate communication with the staff member due to intimidation may result in poor patient outcome

Prevention of Lateral Violence

- Ensure professional accountability
- Provide resources
- Empower staff to confront issues and promote team building
- Provide management support

FAST FACTS in a NUTSHELL

Lateral violence leads to significant financial loss each year due to absenteeism, lack of work performance, and increased turnover.

EMPATHY BURNOUT

Empathy is an emotional connection with a patient. Empathy burnout is the lack of empathy; the ability to feel connected emotionally is no longer there. This type of burnout can impact patient safety.

Impact of Empathy Burnout on Patient Safety

- Stereotyping individuals and then ignoring what they have to say or are feeling
  - Assuming an individual of a certain ethnicity has no pain due to his or her stoic response
  - Concluding that a crying teenager with complaints of abdominal pain is being overly dramatic because of a recent breakup with her boyfriend
- Assigning a lower acuity level due to personal bias, resulting in an inappropriate disposition

Prevention of Empathy Burnout

- When patients are upset or angry, remember that this is a symptom of their situation or illness, not personally directed at you.
- Be aware of your personal bias.
- Take breaks from triage to rejuvenate yourself.
- Work short shifts in triage and rotate to other areas of the department.
- Take time off throughout the year so you can reenergize and best care for others.

Burnout is another term used to describe continued interpersonal and job-related emotional stressors that can influence the overall effectiveness of an organization.

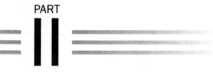

PART

II

Point-of-Entry Processes in Triage Nursing

5

The Patient Arrival

Anna Sivo Montejano

When multiple patients present seeking medical care, the triage nurse determines who is the highest priority. This task can be challenging due to the unpredictable influx of patients at different times of the day. The ability to rapidly assess, determine an initial acuity, and appropriately place patients within the department is imperative to the successful delivery of care. Along with rapid assessment, knowing when to perform a comprehensive assessment and the use of critical thinking skills play a critical role in patient care.

Upon conclusion of this chapter, you will be able to:

1. Define the role of a triage nurse
2. Explain the purpose of a rapid assessment
3. Summarize the data obtained by a comprehensive assessment

ROLES OF A TRIAGE NURSE

A triage nurse's primary role is to identify the sickest patient so treatment may be rendered without delay. Although it seems that this would be the only function, triage nurses wear many hats to fulfill their job on a daily basis. The following examples are additional roles of the triage nurse:

- *Greeter:* Greets patients on arrival and establishes warm friendly environment
- *Resource person:* Problem solver (e.g., wheelchair/cervical spine needs)
- *Department expeditor:* Coordinates placement of patients based on department resources
- *Information center:* Provides information and directions to areas in and around the facility (e.g., radiology, labor and delivery, closest drug store, and bus stop location)

- *Crowd control:* Keeps track of those who are patients versus family and friends
- *Crisis manager:* Handles distraught family member(s), lost belongings, etc.)
- *Safety and security:* Handles the initial contact when an agitated patient needs to be reassured
- *Infection control:* Educates patients about steps that decrease the spread of germs
- *Communicator:* Explains department processes, updates patients/ family
- *Educator:* Educates about first aid, safety issues (helmets), and healthy living
- *Privacy provider:* Provides a private area when needed for stressful situations
- *Reassessment nurse:* Reevaluates patients who are waiting for treatment

RAPID TRIAGE ASSESSMENT

A rapid assessment begins with an across-the-room survey. Visualizing the patient's appearance as he or she enters the facility is the beginning of the rapid assessment. A great deal of information can be gathered by visualizing patients as they step into the waiting room (WR).

- Does the person use a device to assist with ambulation (e.g., cane, walker)?
- Does the facial expression or body language indicate pain?
- What is the skin tone and color?
- Is the gait slow, rapid, or absent?
- Is he or she unresponsive or demonstrating signs of weakness?
- Is there limited eye contact?
- Does the person express fear, anxiety, or agitation?
- Do the clothes give clues to his or her profession (e.g., paint, chemicals, etc.)?

Gathering information on *every* patient who enters the emergency department (ED) is important to assess for a potential or actual life-threatening condition and enable care to be rendered if needed. A few examples of objective information obtained during the rapid assessment include:

- *Airway:* Patent or impaired (e.g., absence of stridor, hoarseness, drooling, facial or oropharyngeal edema)
- *Breathing:* Unlabored or labored (e.g., accessory muscle use, retractions, nasal flaring)
- *Circulation:* Skin color (e.g., pallor, cyanosis) and moisture (e.g., dry, moist, diaphoretic); pulse rate (e.g. fast or slow) and rhythm (e.g. regular or irregular); obvious bleeding

- *Disability (neurological status):* Level of consciousness including Glasgow Coma Scale (GCS) or alert, verbal, pain, unresponsive (AVPU); muscle strength in upper extremities (e.g., pronator drift, grips) and lower extremities (e.g., can the patient lift both legs)

The importance of performing a rapid assessment cannot be over-emphasized. Imagine a scenario in which 10 patients arrive simultaneously to the ED. If the triage nurse performs a lengthy assessment on each individual initially, the last patient in line may be the sickest, with the highest acuity. By rapidly assessing each patient for no more then 60 to 90 seconds, the nurse can *best prioritize* patients, ensuring that higher acuity level patients are seen first.

Delay in Care

If a rapid assessment is not performed as stated previously, delay in recognizing the patient's severity of illness may result in failure to achieve necessary treatment goals or deterioration. The following are examples of situations in which recognition of a high acuity patient may go unnoticed.

- Taking care of patients on a first-come first-serve basis
- Triaging all 10 patients quickly but *maintaining* their original order of arrival when additional information is needed (e.g., comprehensive triage assessment)
- Dismissing the across-the-room assessment
- Allowing bias to hinder the assessment

FAST FACTS in a NUTSHELL

- *Every* patient should have a rapid assessment upon arrival.
- The rapid assessment should be completed by a seasoned nurse. There is so much more to triage than just obtaining the chief complaint.
- Your senses during the rapid assessment may give you a clue about what is going on with the patient (e.g., fruity acetone breath could indicate elevated blood glucose).

IMMEDIATE BEDDING

Immediate bedding is just what it states: providing a bed for a patient immediately upon arrival at the ED as long as specific criteria are first met. In the past, triage was performed as a step-by-step process that required all steps to occur in a specific sequence for the patient to be seen. When the patient arrived at the facility, non–medically trained personnel obtained a chief complaint followed by patient demographic information.

Today, to improve efficiency, safety, and customer service, a parallel process is recommended. A triage nurse should be the first person a patient sees upon arrival at the ED. This nurse has the training, along with the assessment and critical thinking skills, to determine the patient's immediate needs. While the rapid assessment is being performed and the chief complaint obtained, the registration clerk can simultaneously gather the minimal data needed to enter the patient into the system. During this initial encounter, the nurse must assess three criteria to determine the need for immediate bedding (*all three must exist*):

- Obviously ill or injured (*or nurse is able to quickly and confidently determine accurate acuity and appropriate disposition*)
- Open bed (*available or able to obtain*)
- Available care provider(s) (*consider acuity of patient load*) (Triage First, Inc., 2014)

Immediate bedding prevents a patient from being pulled back and forth from the WR to registration, to the WR, to the triage nurse, and so on, getting them where they need to be—an ED bed—so care can be initiated. However, an available care provider (e.g., registered nurse, charge nurse) to accept the patient upon placement in the bed is a critical part of the process.

Points to Consider When Practicing Immediate Bedding

- After a rapid assessment has been completed, follow the immediate bedding criteria.
- If your facility has unlicensed assistive personnel (e.g., patient care technician, nurse's aide, emergency room technician), this staff member would be the ideal choice to escort the patient to a room so the triage nurse can continue triaging. The primary bedside nurse, patient flow coordinator, or charge nurse may also be utilized as a resource for rooming the patient.
  - The triage nurse should remain at triage to identify incoming patients and ensure the safety of patients waiting.
- Ensure proper handoff of the new arrival from the triage nurse to the bedside nurse.
- Once handoff has occurred, the bedside nurse will take over care of the patient.
- When selecting the most appropriate room assignment, consider the acuity level of the bedside nurse's current patients. A high acuity assignment will not allow the bedside nurse to effectively care for the new patient arrival.

If bed availability increases at a time when an influx of lower acuity patients arrive, the triage nurse may consider placing a patient in a bed even though he or she does not meet the first immediate bedding criteria, "obviously injured or sick." However, it is important to avoid overwhelming the main ED beds, thus eliminating availability for higher acuity patients who may arrive.

===*FAST FACTS in a NUTSHELL*

- A rapid assessment is used to identify high acuity patients and initiate immediate bedding criteria when indicated.
- A patient may arrive with airway, breathing, circulation, and neurological status intact, but some aspect of their presentation (e.g., white particles on clothing) may give you a clue to an exposure that requires immediate isolation to protect other patients and the staff.
- If a patient states that he or she was involved in a bus accident, explosion, or similar incident, be prepared to initiate a facility disaster response; other patients may be arriving soon. Follow your protocol!

COMPREHENSIVE TRIAGE ASSESSMENT

The comprehensive assessment follows the rapid assessment and supplies the remainder of the patient's history so that a final acuity level can be determined. *On average,* a comprehensive triage should take 2 to 5 minutes; however, there may be times when this process takes longer.

Reasons for a Longer Comprehensive Triage Assessment

- Elderly patient (e.g., delay in motor movement, responds slowly to questions, hard of hearing)
- Patient with numerous medication bottles
- Language barrier
- Patient with multiple layers of clothing
- Patient safety issue (e.g., psychiatric)
- Child who requires an antipyretic
- Confused or uncooperative patient

Not all patients will receive a comprehensive assessment at triage. When a bed is available and immediate bedding criteria met, the comprehensive triage will occur at the bedside. With the patient in the room the physician and nurse can simultaneously hear the history and partake in the physical assessment. This process is efficient and decreases the questioning that the patient experiences.

Information Obtained During the Comprehensive Triage Assessment

- Vital signs
- Weight and height
- Complete history (e.g., medical, surgical, etc.)
- Medications
- Allergies to medications and foods
- Screening questions (e.g., domestic violence, fall risk, etc.)

When obtaining the comprehensive assessment, completing the history while simultaneously obtaining the vital signs can save time. Asking for the medication list can help the nurse with information regarding the medical history. For example, when patients are asked about their medical history, they may state only that they have diabetes. However, when specifically asked about medications, a patient may provide information about three medications he or she is taking: an antihypertensive, a lipid-lowering agent, and an oral hypoglycemic. Upon further questioning, the patient may confirm, "Oh yes, I do have high cholesterol and high blood pressure." When the patient is questioned about medications *before* the medical history, this delay in information can be prevented.

FAST FACTS in a NUTSHELL

- In some facilities two or more nurses work in the triage area. One nurse should focus on the rapid assessment while another nurse should complete the comprehensive assessment. Stress the importance of one rapid triage nurse that knows all the patients.
- During busy hours, if the rapid assessment nurse has no incoming patients to assess, he or she may assist the comprehensive nurse.
- If comprehensive assessments are consistently taking a long time, there may be a breakdown in the process or resources (e.g., lack of support, supplies), or both
- In facilities where there is only one triage nurse, this nurse will perform the rapid triage assessments and, when time allows, complete a comprehensive triage assessment. If

you are performing a comprehensive triage assessment and additional patients have arrived:

- Stop the triage, kindly excusing yourself
- Rapidly assess the incoming patient(s)
- Return to complete the comprehensive triage assessment

CRITICAL THINKING SKILLS

Critical thinking is used every minute in triage as the nurse assesses patients upon their arrival. As nurses, we use our senses of sight, smell, hearing, and touch while asking questions to gather information. Once the information is gathered, we then critically think, synthesizing the information obtained to determine an accurate acuity level.

Examples of Critical Thinking

- Are the patient's history and medications contributing to the signs and symptoms he or she is exhibiting?
- Is there information that the patient may not be sharing that requires further probing?
- Are illegal substances causing or escalating the signs and symptoms of the patient's complaint?
- Does what the patient is telling you make sense?
- Has someone accompanied the patient, and is that person having an impact on how much the patient is telling you?
  - For example, a 15-year-old who is complaining of abdominal pain may not disclose that she is pregnant because her mother is sitting next to her.

Intuition is based less on evidence-based practice than on the experiences of the nurse. Some of the phrases used to describe this instinctive feeling are "a gut feeling," "instinct," and "a sixth sense." It can be hard for a seasoned nurse to explain these responses to a novice nurse because they operate outside of conscious reasoning. Novice nurses want to know, "How did you know?", when all the nurse can answer is, "I just had a feeling." This ability comes from knowledge and experience.

Examples of a Nurse's Intuition

- The nurse moves a patient with a simple bee sting to a room in front of the nurse's station to be monitored.
  - Twenty minutes later the patient has a cardiac arrest.

- An unkempt female patient arrives via ambulance with abdominal pain and diarrhea. Medics and staff downplay the scenario.
  - One hour later the nurse has an uneasy feeling and looks under the patient's sheet, a newborn baby has arrived.
- A psychiatric patient has been experiencing seizures while awake. Medical staff attribute the seizures to her psychiatric history, and no computed tomography (CT) scan is ordered.
  - The nurse assesses several neurological deficits and advocates for ordering a CT scan of the brain. The patient's diagnosis after the CT scan: malignant brain tumor.

FAST FACTS in a NUTSHELL

Intuition can save someone's life. Making a decision without relying on intuition can result in a poor outcome.

REFERENCE

Triage First, Inc. (2014). *ED triage: Comprehensive course.* Asheville, NC: Author.

6

Customer Service in Triage Nursing

Lynn Sayre Visser

In health care today, patient satisfaction is more important than ever. Patient satisfaction is linked not only to high-quality clinical care but to customer service as well. The success of an organization depends on its customers; thus, staff should recognize that both real and perceived experiences impact a person's impression of the service rendered. Since you never get a second chance to make a first impression, making that first interaction a positive experience is essential. Staff training in the delivery of top-notch service is a key element to creating a customer-friendly environment that promotes patient satisfaction. However, no amount of training will enhance the delivery of service for disgruntled staff. Thus, first and foremost, staff must be cared for. Happy staff = Happy patients!

Upon conclusion of this chapter, you will be able to:

1. State two key elements of providing effective customer service
2. List two examples of the right words at the right time
3. Explain the importance of rounding and reassessments in the waiting room
4. Discuss service recovery efforts

PROVIDING EFFECTIVE CUSTOMER SERVICE

Care for Staff First

Customer service does not come easily to all staff, especially unhappy staff. Staff members must first feel *valued* and *cared for* before being asked to deliver excellent service. Staff who are satisfied with their work environment can more easily convey a sense of caring in a genuine tone of voice and with corresponding body language. Thus,

45

measures should be taken to build staff camaraderie and address workplace issues. Consider whether the following issues exist:

- The presence of lateral violence on the unit that needs to be addressed (see Chapter 4 for additional information)
- Staff who are suffering from compassion fatigue or empathy burnout
- The absence of regular breaks and mealtimes
- Lack of support from the management team
- Staff who do not feel their input is valued or considered
- The absence of or limited teamwork
- Lack of adequate supplies and resources available to function effectively

Tackling issues like these must occur first and *then* customer service training can follow.

Since the triage nurse often sets the tone for the patient experience, special consideration should be given to the unique needs of the staff working in the triage area. The triage nurse needs to maintain positive energy while utilizing critical thinking skills; thus, rest breaks are essential. If your facility is not doing these things already, consider implementation of the following:

- A break nurse or a systematic plan to ensure the triage nurse receives regular rest, meal, and bathroom breaks
- Shorter shifts in triage (e.g., 4 or 6 hours)

Most individuals find maintaining a welcoming smile and positive attitude for an entire 12-hour triage shift to be extremely difficult; thus, shorter shifts at triage are encouraged.

Positive Staff Recognition

Programs that encourage other staff, patients, or visitors to acknowledge a person who delivers exceptional service are recommended. Recognition for a job well done praises the meaningful work, encourages a person to repeat the positive behavior, and promotes a healthier work environment. In addition, the *purpose* behind the work is celebrated. The recognition can be given to a staff member caught in the act of delivering top-notch care, having a heartfelt interaction with a patient or family member, or going above and beyond expected service. Ideas for recognizing others include:

- Use of a "hot compliments" board where others (e.g., patients, visitors, or staff) can share positive words about one staff member or the team as a whole

- "Caught ya" cards (e.g., movie tickets, coffee card, handwritten note) that are immediately given to a staff member caught in the act of providing exceptional service
- Posting positive patient satisfaction survey comments or letters from patients and family members where staff can view them
- Sending a personal, handwritten note to the home of the staff member

Honoring one staff member at a time builds team cohesiveness, supports a positive work environment, and encourages other staff to recognize the excellent work of their colleagues. In time, every team member will make the effort to acknowledge others. Only one person is needed to begin the process of creating a happier, healthier work environment. Is that staff member you?

Training for Service Excellence

Upon initiating customer service training, staff should gain a clear understanding of who their customers are. Customers in a health care facility extend far beyond the patient to encompass visitors, physicians, other employees, pharmaceutical representatives, and even the pizza delivery person, to name just a few. The emergency department (ED) is often the hospital point-of-entry; thus, the triage team interacts with many individuals entering the facility. Customer service training should include:

- Understanding the difference between customers and patients
- Scripting during key moments of truth (e.g., lost patient belongings or lab specimen)
- Service recovery efforts (e.g., rectifying a poor experience)

Giving staff the tools needed to deliver excellent customer service is essential. Training can occur via the following:

- A formalized live program with lecture and discussion
- Self-paced online education
- Simulation training with case scenarios
- Observation of staff who frequently receive positive comments

Customer service training needs to include team members throughout the continuum of care. Anyone who comes in contact with customers or patients within the facility requires training. Included in this group are:

- Direct care providers (e.g., registered nurses, licensed vocational/practical nurses, medical providers, paramedics, unlicensed personnel, etc.)

- Ancillary staff including radiology, laboratory, dietary, security, and environmental services
- Administrative team members
- Volunteers

SCRIPTING

Scripting is a common catchword in health care today. You may be thinking, why scripting? Do I really need to be told what to say? Chances are you do an excellent job in responding to questions. However, having *the right words at the most appropriate time* can make the difference in meeting patient and family needs; thus, having a few scripts available that can address certain situations is important. Scripting helps customers feel positive about the service received and has been shown to decrease the frequency with which patients leave before being seen by a medical provider. The scenarios that follow are examples of common situations that arise in triage settings. Many other scripts can be developed that speak to the needs of common questions and concerns of your customers.

Wait Times

Scenario: An ambulatory patient who arrives at your facility encounters a waiting room (WR) with standing room only. As the triage nurse, you can anticipate the patient's first question.

- *The question:* How long will I have to wait?
- *What you may be thinking:* Don't you see the 50 people sitting in the WR and lying on the floor? Didn't you hear the sirens and see the three ambulances that pulled up when you did? At the rate patients are arriving, you may wait 6, 8, or maybe even 12 hours.
- *Why you don't say what you are thinking:* Giving information about long wait times could be interpreted as coercion. Encouraging a patient to leave before receiving a medical screening exam (MSE) can lead to an Emergency Medical Treatment and Active Labor Act (EMTALA) violation costing the facility a $50,000 fine. (See Chapter 7 for additional information.)
- *A good response:* "I wish I could give you a time, but it depends on so many factors. Patients are not seen in the order of arrival but rather based on the severity of their condition, with potentially life-threatening conditions given the highest priority. If someone arrives in active labor, they will be seen first." Often, lower acuity patients who believe their medical condition is a high priority understand that a woman in labor will be a higher treatment priority. Providing this example eliminates all lower acuity presentations (including those of women, men, the elderly, and children) and is rarely disputed by the waiting patient!

Directions

Scenario: A man arrives at ED triage looking for his wife, who has been transferred to the intensive care unit (ICU).

- *The question:* How do I get to the ICU?
- *What you may be thinking:* Does this man really think I have time to explain directions? I have 10 people waiting to be triaged!
- *Why you don't say what you are thinking:* The work you have to do is the least of this man's concerns because his wife is critically ill.
- *A good response:* "Let me get someone to escort you so we can get you to your wife as quickly as possible." Escorting people to their destination gives a feeling of caring and compassion and lessens anxiety during times of stress.

Drinks

Scenario: A woman arrives complaining of left upper quadrant pain after a fall from a bicycle.

- *The question:* Can I have a cup of water while I wait?
- *What you may be thinking:* Nope! Absolutely not! No way! I see a potential surgery in your future!
- *Why you don't say what you are thinking:* Simply giving an answer of "no" to a patient comes off as rude and insensitive.
- *A good response:* "I would love to get you a glass of water once we make sure your symptoms are not too serious. Your health is our top priority." Patients appreciate your concern for them, and an explanation of *why* they should not drink fluid is important.

Status Improves While Waiting

Scenario: Parents arrive with a child who has a temperature of 104 °F (40 °C). Acetaminophen is given at triage and the parents and child wait to be seen by a provider. While waiting, the temperature decreases to 100.1 °F (38.4 °C).

- *The question:* My son is feeling better so I am thinking about taking him home and seeing his pediatrician tomorrow. What do you think?
- *What you may be thinking:* The kid looks fine, acts fine, and if he were mine, I would want to take him home, too!
- *Why you don't say what you are thinking:* You never want to downplay a patient condition. If the parents take the child home before the MSE and the child has a seizure, unidentified meningitis, or

other concerning diagnosis, the child may have a poor outcome posing a serious liability risk to both you and the facility.

- *A good response:* "I am glad he is feeling better, but I would really like to have him seen by a medical provider so we can make sure the cause of the fever is nothing of concern. I will feel better if we get him checked out and I bet you will, too."

COMMUNICATION

Communication is an essential component in making customers happy. People presenting to triage are seeking information and answers to medical signs and symptoms. Providing information in terms that are understandable to the individual is critical. Some facilities hand out an "itinerary" upon the patient's arrival that sets the tone for the visit. The itinerary may include:

- An explanation of realistic expectations for the visit
- Rationale of why a first-come, first-served system is not utilized
- Explanations regarding wait times
- Purpose of a medical provider in triage
- When and how diagnostic testing may occur
- Why patients move between different rooms and departments
- A signature from each staff member delivering care (e.g., nurses, medical providers, unlicensed personnel, etc.)

Consider handing out business cards to your patients or their family members. Many facilities will not pay for employee business cards, but this practice is something you can do to go the extra mile. The initials after your name are often a great conversation piece with patients and visitors, especially if you hold a national certification in your area of specialty.

FAST FACTS in a NUTSHELL

- Be aware that simply saying the correct words means nothing if the nonverbal communication does not match the spoken words.
- Do not read from a script word for word. Rather, know the key ideas of the script and deliver the message in your own words with emotion and sincerity.
- Provide information and reassurance!

ROUNDING

Rounding in the WR should be a routine element of caring for patients. Depending on the facility, the role may be filled by the triage nurse, charge nurse, unlicensed personnel, or a patient advocate team member. Rounding can include:

• Checking for WR cleanliness
• Seeking answers to questions for patients and family members
• Ensuring magazines are available and the television is set to age-appropriate channels
• Increasing awareness of individuals in the WR (e.g., knowing who are the patients and who the visitors are, since you may find someone who is seeking care and never got registered, did not receive a rapid assessment on arrival, etc.)
• Providing a verbal update to those waiting regarding the status of the department (e.g., ED patient admissions going to the in-patient floor soon, additional staff just came on shift, etc.)

Some staff are not comfortable speaking loudly above the WR crowd. Additionally, the layout of the WR may make a one-time announcement difficult for all to hear. Regardless of the situation, communication with those waiting is imperative. Addressing multiple small groups of people can be effective, as well. Many people in the WR fear the unknown. The unknown could be a diagnosis, the facility process, or the wait time. Be creative. The point is to *communicate* with those in the WR and let them know you care.

REASSESSMENTS

Prolonged wait times can lead to changes in a patient presentation. The importance of reassessments utilizing critical thinking, guidelines (see Chapter 8), and the facility policy cannot be overstated. Reassessments may include:

• Vital signs
• Pain assessment
• Determining effectiveness of previously administered medication (e.g., fever control following acetaminophen or ibuprofen, blood glucose level after orange juice is given for hypoglycemia, pain level after an oral analgesic is administered)

Reassessment provides an additional opportunity to update patients about their status, answer questions, and give additional reassurance. Many nurses feel overwhelmed at triage and the thought of reassessing waiting patients seems impossible. However, measures to safeguard patient safety while limiting personal liability at triage are essential. Develop a facility plan to support reassessments and their completion per policy.

FAST FACTS in a NUTSHELL

- Patients assigned a mid-level acuity (e.g., Emergency Severity Index or Canadian Triage Acuity Scale level 3) who wait for treatment may experience a change in medical condition. When a change in the patient's medical condition goes unnoticed, rapid deterioration may occur. Therefore, ongoing reassessment of waiting patients is critical!
- Do not let your guard down with any waiting patient!

SERVICE RECOVERY

Service recovery programs are vital when an interaction with a customer takes an undesirable turn. Staff should quickly and honestly identify the patient or visitor having a poor experience and take measures to make things better. Sometimes bringing another staff member into the situation to explain the mishap can be helpful. Owning up to an error, whether you were personally responsible for the mistake or not, can be extremely difficult to do. However, the reality is that health care is a service industry; thus, creating positive customer experiences is essential.

Negative Customer Experiences

Service recovery may be needed in circumstances like the following:

- The patient misunderstood the wait time frames and plan of care
- The patient's blood tests were lost in transit to the lab
- The required diagnostic x-ray was never ordered
- The triage nurse stated he or she would return to the WR to escort the family member to the patient but failed to return

Negative customer experiences should be seen as an opportunity. Steps can be taken to address the following:

- Process failures
- Communication hurdles
- Misunderstandings

Maintaining a service recovery log book and reflecting on the experiences and service recovery efforts can provide good information for future problem resolution. Does the same problem occur on the same shift routinely? Are family members always left to linger in the WR due to lack of staff who can escort them to their loved one? Efforts to identify patterns where service recovery was required should be made so the root cause can be addressed.

Resolving the Negative Experience

First and foremost, the error or negative experience should be resolved as soon as possible. In the event blood tests were lost in transit to the lab, the patient's blood specimen should be redrawn as rapidly as possible and hand delivered to the lab. After a sincere apology by the staff member, an additional service recovery effort can be initiated and may include:

- Providing a free meal in the cafeteria
- Delivering flowers to the patient's hospital room or home
- Giving a small gift card that can be used at the cafeteria or gift shop
- Acknowledgment from the charge nurse or management team
- Follow-up phone call the next day

EVALUATING SERVICE EXCELLENCE EFFORTS

Reflecting on customer service practices and efforts should be ongoing in every facility. Gathering benchmark data regarding service delivery efforts before, during, and after customer service training is important. This evaluation should occur both continually and at frequent, regular intervals. Comparing benchmark data during different time frames reveals information about attainment of pre-identified metric goals and helps determine areas for improvement. Processes that enhance patient safety and patient satisfaction often improve staff satisfaction. The cycle of happier staff resulting in happier patients leads to a better environment for all.

Legal Concerns in Triage Nursing

Deb Jeffries

Emergency health care is saturated with potential legal pitfalls that are nowhere more obvious than during the emergency department (ED) triage process. The triage nurse must be knowledgeable about a vast array of clinical presentations; be able to think critically; and rapidly and accurately prioritize incoming patients—all while maintaining excellent customer service skills. In addition to this abbreviated list of triage nurse qualifications, the nurse must be knowledgeable about the legal expectations of ED triage. These expectations stem from governmental bodies and regulatory agencies such as the state board of nursing. The individual nurse must know what these requirements are, as defined by these entities, before a challenging situation arises.

Upon conclusion of this chapter, you will be able to:

1. State governmental and regulatory requirements affecting ED triage
2. Identify patient's rights regarding privacy and consent
3. Discuss high-risk legal considerations at triage

EMERGENCY MEDICAL TREATMENT AND ACTIVE LABOR ACT (EMTALA)

EMTALA, known as the "anti-dumping statute," was enacted in 1986 as part of the Consolidated Omnibus Budget Reconciliation Act of 1985 (COBRA). Often referred to as the "unfunded federal mandate," EMTALA responded to an ugly chapter in the history of emergency care in the United States: the "dumping" of the poor and often disenfranchised onto public hospitals. As a result of these actions by individual hospitals and staff, some patients died and poor fetal outcomes occurred as people were turned away from a handful of EDs due to inability to pay. Out of this context, EMTALA was born. EMTALA mandates that every patient receive:

- A medical screening exam (MSE)
- Necessary stabilizing medical treatment
- An appropriate transfer to a higher level of care if necessary

Who Can Perform a Medical Screening Exam?

EMTALA legislation allows for a physician or a qualified medical person, identified by the facility, to perform the MSE.

Qualified Medical Person (QMP)

- The hospital must formally determine who can perform the MSE
- This must be defined in a document approved by the governing board of the hospital
- Those designated must be identified in the hospital by-laws or in rules and regulations governing the medical staff
- It is *not* acceptable for the medical director to make informal designations of who may perform the MSE (Centers for Medicare and Medicaid Services [CMS], 2010, 2012)

EMTALA does not specifically define (outside of the conscripts just discussed) who can perform the MSE.

> A hospital must formally determine who is qualified to perform the initial medical screening examinations, i.e., qualified medical person. While it is permissible for a hospital to designate a non-physician practitioner as the qualified medical person, the designated non-physician practitioner must be set forth in a document that is approved by the governing board of the hospital. (CMS, 2012, p. 5)

FAST FACTS in a NUTSHELL

- According to the CMS, the MSE is anything and everything that is necessary to determine whether or not the patient has an emergency medical condition (EMC).
- An EMC is any presentation with acute symptoms of *sufficient severity* that if medical care was not provided that the patient (including those not yet born) would be at risk for serious injury or death. Symptoms of sufficient severity includes *pain*.

EMTALA Pitfalls

Most ED triage nurses realize that EMTALA means that every person seeking medical care at an ED in the United States has the rights presented in this chapter. A few other stipulations include:

- Accurate documentation should be initiated for every person who presents for care, including patients who decide not to remain for treatment
- A potential EMTALA violation exists if you *suggest* that a patient should seek care elsewhere
- Federal law (EMTALA) supersedes state law every time
- EMTALA applies to every hospital that has a dedicated ED and accepts Medicare funding
- Signs must be posted informing patients of their rights
- Signs must be provided in language(s) most common to the community seeking care
- Hospital property includes the area within 250 yards of the building (CMS, 2010, 2012).

=============================*FAST FACTS in a NUTSHELL*

- *Scenario:* A child is brought to the ED by a parent because of a runny nose, ear pain, and fever. The child is in no acute distress. The triage nurse tells the parent, "Your child is doing very well, you may not be aware of this, but there is a pediatric urgent care just across the street. Your child will be seen more quickly there."
- You cannot suggest that patients seek care elsewhere. This is an EMTALA violation.
- The medical screening exam or treatment *should never be delayed* to inquire about the patient's ability to pay.

CONSENT TO TREATMENT

Knowing the laws and requirements that are applicable in your facility is imperative. There are four types of consent:

- *Expressed consent:* A competent person gives consent for treatment.
- *Implied consent:* Threat to life or limb exists and the person is unable to give consent.

- *Involuntary consent*: An incompetent person refuses to consent. Competence is determined by a medical provider based on a variety of factors. Our responsibility is to thoroughly document the subjective and objective data and all interactions with the patient. *Documentation is critical!*
- *Informed consent*: Consent is given by a competent individual for a specific procedure. In some jurisdictions this consent is to be obtained by a physician.

Competent patients who are of an age and circumstance at which they can consent to treatment have the right to determine what care they will receive (Emergency Nurses Association [ENA], 2007, 2010, 2013).

Special Considerations Regarding Consent

Scenario: A 16-year-old girl presents to triage requesting treatment for a sexually transmitted disease but does not want her parents notified. Does she have the right to consent for her own treatment?

In most states the answer is "yes." However, you must be certain of the laws regarding minors seeking care for themselves. In many states minors are allowed to seek care if it relates to pregnancy, sexually transmitted diseases, substance abuse, and methods of birth control. However, the age of consent varies from state to state and country to country. Minors who are legally emancipated may consent for their own care. Emancipation rules vary by area, so be familiar with the requirements where you practice.

FAST FACTS in a NUTSHELL

You are responsible for knowing the applicable laws in your state or country as well as corresponding policies at the facility in which you practice.

LWT, LWBS, LPMSE, LBTC, AMA

These acronyms are just a few that are bandied about when discussing patients who leave before they are discharged home by a provider. These terms are *not* synonymous:

- *Left without treatment (LWT):* May occur before or after triage
- *Left without being seen (LWBS):* Patient leaves after triage but before seeing a provider
- *Left prior to the MSE (LPMSE):* May occur before or after triage but before the MSE is initiated

- *Left before treatment complete (LBTC)*: Patients who leave after treatment initiated by the provider but before formal disposition
- *Against medical advice (AMA)*: Patients who leave against the advice of the provider (a subset of LBTC). By definition, this refers only to those who have been advised of the risk associated with leaving and who choose to leave regardless of those risks (Welch et al., 2011).

Although many factors influence a patient's decision to stay or leave, two of the most significant factors are the wait time and communication (or lack thereof). Certain characteristics exist that are consistent among those who leave; these include:

- Male gender
- Low socioeconomic status
- Low urgency, low acuity
- African American race

Almost half of those who leave would stay if comfort measures had been offered (Johnson, Myers, Wineholt, Pollack, & Kusmierz, 2009; Vierheller, 2013).

When a person leaves before the MSE is completed, an increased risk for a poor patient outcome exists. According to one study, approximately half of those who leave without being seen by a provider seek care elsewhere in the following 24 hours (Vierheller, 2013). Every effort must be made to encourage patients to stay, even when the department is at maximum capacity and the staff feel overwhelmed. When patients communicate that they want to leave, sometimes a simple inquiry as to *why* they want to leave can provide enough information to address the specific issue.

Remember, you absolutely *cannot* suggest to patients that they should seek care elsewhere, and under EMTALA a log of *all* patients who present to the ED for care must be recorded regardless of whether they choose to stay. Our responsibility begins the moment that we become aware that the patient is seeking emergency care. The fact that a person has not yet received an MSE does *not* change our responsibility or the fact that the person is a patient!

HEALTH INSURANCE PORTABILITY AND ACCOUNTABILITY ACT (HIPAA)

HIPAA—the Health Insurance Portability and Accountability Act of 1996—is another federal mandate. So much of what we have heard since 1996 regarding HIPAA is not about the mainstay of the legislation, which was designed to combat health care fraud and abuse, but about the requirements to protect and ensure patient confidentiality in regard to *any individually identifiable health information*. This practice is known as "protecting personal health information (PHI)" (ENA, 2010, 2013). Protecting this information can be daunting during the triage process, and many ED nurses have the perception that it is not only difficult but rather impossible. This perception comes from a distorted view that confidentiality is based upon physical plant parameters when, instead, body behavior and actions of the individual obtaining the information are the driving factors.

Meeting HIPAA Privacy Requirements

We can meet HIPAA privacy requirements when interacting with patients by doing the following:

- Lowering our voices
- Moving physically closer to the patient
- When necessary, asking the patient to take a few steps away from others (including those accompanying them)

Although this is effective most the time, there may be instances when we do have to inquire about the reason for the visit within the potential hearing of another. For example, as we immediately expedite the care of an individual arriving by private vehicle who is cyanotic with altered level of consciousness another person *might* overhear an inquiry directed toward obtaining information from the patient's family. Our responsibility to patients and their families is to ensure *patient safety* through the initiation of any necessary immediate interventions. Every possible effort to maintain patient confidentiality should occur, but we cannot compromise patient safety.

FAST FACTS in a NUTSHELL

When in doubt about legal issues, call risk management.

REPORTABLE CONDITIONS AND EVENTS

Although reportable conditions and events vary from one jurisdiction to another, knowing what is reportable and what is not in your geographical area is imperative to your role as the triage nurse. Commonly reportable conditions in most states include:

- Elder abuse
- Sexual assault and rape
- Suicide

- Assault with weapons
- Stab wounds
- Injury from explosives
- Homicide
- Sexually transmitted infections
- Child abuse
- Certain communicable diseases (e.g., tuberculosis)
- Gunshot wounds
- Injury, death, or illness from a medical device

What is important to note is that privacy laws do not apply to legally defined reportable conditions or events. For example, if a patient presents to the ED with a gunshot wound and the triage nurse calls local law enforcement and provides the patient's name, address, and date of birth, the nurse has *not* committed a HIPAA violation by providing protected patient information, because this event is a reportable condition.

REFERENCES

Centers for Medicare and Medicaid Services. (2010). *CMS manual system Pub. 100-07 State operations provider certification.* Retrieved January 18, 2014, from http://www.cms.gov/Regulations-and-Guidance/Guidance/Transmittals/downloads/R60SOMA.pdf

Centers for Medicare and Medicaid Services. (2012). *State operations manual Appendix V–Interpretive guidelines–Responsibilities of medicare participating hospitals in emergency cases.* Retrieved January 18, 2014, from http://www.cms.gov/Regulations-and-Guidance/Guidance/Manuals/Downloads/som107ap_v_emerg.pdf

Emergency Nurses Association. (2007). *Emergency nursing core curriculum* (6th ed.). St. Louis, MO: Saunders.

Emergency Nurses Association. (2010). *Sheehy's emergency nursing principles and practice.* St. Louis, MO: Mosby.

Emergency Nurses Association. (2013). *Sheehy's manual of emergency care* (7th ed.). St. Louis, MO: Mosby.

Johnson, M., Myers, S., Wineholt, J., Pollack, M., & Kusmierz, A. L. (2009). Patients who leave the emergency department without being seen. *Journal of Emergency Nursing, 35*(2), 105–108.

Vierheller, C. C. (2013). Evaluating left without being seen and against medical advice departures in a rural emergency department. *Journal of Emergency Nursing, 39*(1), 67–71.

Welch, S. J., Asplin, B. R., Stone-Griffith, S., Davidson, S. J., Augustine, J., & Schuur, J. (2011). Emergency department operational metrics, measures and definitions: Results of the Second Performance Measures and Benchmarking Summit. *Annals of Emergency Medicine, 58*(1), 33–40.

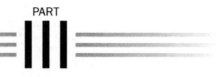

PART

III

Nursing Essentials
for Effective Triage

8

Triage Acuity Scales

Deb Jeffries

A triage acuity level refers to the potential severity of a patient's illness or injury. Assigning a correct acuity level is one of the most important responsibilities of the triage nurse, because the prioritization of the patient determines and sets the trajectory of care for the entire patient stay. Therefore, the acuity level assigned must be an accurate reflection of the patient's condition at the time of triage. The goal of all triage acuity scales is to appropriately and accurately determine priority of care. This chapter introduces the more commonly used triage acuity scales including the Emergency Severity Index (ESI), Canadian Triage and Acuity Scale (CTAS), Australasian Triage Scale (ATS), and Manchester Triage System (MTS).

Upon conclusion of this chapter, you will be able to:

1. Understand the significance of standardization of triage acuity scales
2. Identify three factors that lead to mistriage
3. List four commonly used triage acuity scales

TRIAGE ACUITY: OVERVIEW

Emergency departments (EDs) have historically used triage acuity scales or rating systems that were highly subjective, with little to no research as to their reliability and validity. For many years most EDs used a 3-level triage acuity scale, typically categorizing patients as:

- Emergent
- Urgent
- Non-urgent

This approach to prioritization worked for patients who fell clearly into one of those categories, such as the severely hypotensive and tachycardic patient with an upper gastrointestinal bleeding (obviously emergent) or the patient without a physical complaint presenting for a medication refill (obviously non-urgent). However, a patient with a suspicion of acute coronary syndrome who was pain free would receive an urgent acuity level on a 3-level scale, because he or she could not possibly have the same acuity level as a patient who was obviously clinically unstable (e.g., an unresponsive patient) (Triage First, Inc., 2013).

Historically nurses also lacked formal education related to the use of acuity scales. This lack of education was not isolated to acuity scales but extended to the triage process as a whole. Unfortunately, in some facilities just having a nursing license was a sufficient qualification to be assigned to the triage role. *Regardless of the specific triage acuity scale used, nurses must receive comprehensive education regarding the appropriate use of that scale.* Use of a valid and reliable 5-level triage acuity scale provides more discrimination between acuity levels, compared to the days of the 3-level scales, and allows the nurse to more appropriately determine who can and cannot wait for care. Table 8.1 demonstrates the variations noted among systems. Many other scales also exist worldwide.

FAST FACTS in a NUTSHELL

- Nurses providing care at the stretcher-side can attest to the complexity of the patients seen in most EDs today. For the triage nurse, assigning the correct acuity level is first and foremost a patient safety issue.
- Assigning a correct acuity level can help staff obtain the resources needed to provide appropriate and effective patient care. However, this can only be a reality if we use a common language that communicates to strategic leaders how sick the patients really are.

TABLE 8.1 Comparing Triage Systems

Level	5- Level Systems	4-Level Systems	3-Level Systems	2-Level Systems
1	Resuscitation	Life-threatening		
2	Emergent	Emergent	Emergent	Emergent
3	Urgent	Urgent	Urgent	
4	Nonurgent	Nonurgent	Nonurgent	Nonemergent
5	Referred			

Source: Buettner (2013).

MISTRIAGE

Mistriage is the assigning of a triage acuity level that is higher or lower than is warranted.

What Causes Mistriage?

A number of factors contribute to mistriage, including:

- Lack of education
- Inexperience
- Empathy burnout (Triage First, Inc., 2013)

Avoiding Mistriage

Mistriage can be avoided by ensuring that:

- Nurses are educated in the triage process and the specific acuity scale being used
- Only experienced, educated nurses are assigned to the triage role
- Only the scale-specific criteria are used when determining acuity (Agency for Healthcare Research and Quality, 2012)

══════════════════════════════*FAST FACTS in a NUTSHELL*

Although assigning either a higher or a lower acuity level than is indicated for the patient is mistriage, it is unlikely that the patient will be harmed by selecting the higher level. However, the patient can potentially be harmed by choosing the lower level. Triage nurses should use a valid and reliable 5-level triage acuity scale and always act with the best interest of the patient in mind.

SPECIFIC TRIAGE ACUITY SCALES

The following discussion is a brief introduction to the more commonly used triage scales, including ESI, CTAS, ATS, and MTS. The intricate details of each triage scale cannot be covered in the limited number of pages contained in this book. To use these scales effectively, additional comprehensive training is required.

Emergency Severity Index (ESI)

The ESI is a well-researched 5-level triage acuity scale with strong inter-rater reliability that is used extensively in the United States as well as in other countries. As it is an algorithm-driven scale, the nurse begins with every patient as a *potential* level 1 acuity and then moves down the algorithm when the patient does not meet specific criteria. For lower level acuities, ESI involves considering the number of resources (e.g., x-rays, laboratory tests, electrocardiograms, etc.) that the patient requires for the provider to make a disposition based upon what is "prudent and customary" care (Gilboy, Tanabe, Travers, & Rosenau, 2011, p. 32) as well as danger zone vital signs. ESI encompasses both adult and pediatric presentations in *The Emergency Severity Index (ESI): A Triage Tool for Emergency Department Care, Version 4. Implementation Handbook 2012 Edition*. (This handbook can be obtained from the Agency for Healthcare Research and Quality by calling 1-800-358-9295 or by e-mailing AHRQPubs@ahrq.hhs.gov. A downloaded version of the handbook can be obtained online at www.ahrq.gov.)

Canadian Triage and Acuity Scale (CTAS)

CTAS is also a well-researched 5-level triage acuity scale used worldwide for both adult and pediatric patient populations. This scale allows for the assigning of acuity based upon chief complaint and associated signs and symptoms along with the consideration of modifiers.

Modifiers are physiological and subjective considerations and are classified as either first order (e.g., vital signs, pain severity, mechanism of injury), which apply to many complaints, or second order (e.g., hypoglycemia), which are more specifically related to fewer complaints. This acuity scale provides reassessment time frame guidelines. CTAS implementation guidelines and subsequent revisions can be obtained from www.caep.ca/resources/ctas#support.

Australasian Triage Scale (ATS)

The ATS is a valid and reliable 5-category scale that is used in New Zealand and Australia. This scale was developed with the goal of matching the patient's clinical urgency with timelines of care by considering how long a patient should wait for assessment and treatment from the time of his or her arrival. The ATS uses a conceptual question to drive the acuity designation by asking, "This patient should wait for medical assessment and treatment no longer than. . ." (Australasian College for Emergency Medicine, 2013a, p. 1). Clinical descriptors assist the nurse in determining the acuity level. For example, some category 1 clinical descriptors include:

- Cardiac or respiratory arrest, or both
- Imminent risk to airway
- Blood pressure less than 80 mmHg in adults

- Child or infant in severe shock
- Extreme respiratory distress
- Unresponsive or responds to pain only
  (Australasian College for Emergency Medicine, 2013b)

Additional information regarding the use of the ATS can be accessed at www.acem.org.au and www.health.gov.au.

Manchester Triage System (MTS)

The MTS is a valid and reliable 5-level triage acuity scale widely used in Europe and the United Kingdom. This acuity system uses an algorithm approach with over 50 detailed flow charts. An example of a flow chart can be viewed at http://tinyurl.com/mw4qhqr. The triage nurse chooses a category based upon the patient's presenting complaint. The nurse then makes the acuity decision based upon signs and symptoms, also known as discriminators, as they relate to the flow chart chosen. General discriminators can be viewed at http://tinyurl.com/pvvnn6f. The MTS core text by the Manchester Triage Group (2014) provides additional information about this acuity scale (see the reference at the end of this chapter).

===*FAST FACTS in a NUTSHELL*

Not all patients fit into our nice, neat acuity categories. However, when the acuity scale criteria are used, most of the time you will be able to determine the appropriate acuity level.

A Few Final Thoughts

As noted earlier, this survey of the 5-level triage acuity scale is merely a brief introduction. *Any* emergency nurse with the responsibility of assigning an acuity designation must be thoroughly familiar with the specific criteria of the scale being used. To accomplish this, *education is a must.*

Another often-debated issue surrounding triage acuity designations is whether, once assigned, the triage acuity should be changed based upon a change in patient status or because a colleague disagrees with the original acuity assigned. The answer to this question is a resounding "*No!*" Once assigned, the original triage acuity *does not change.* (Hint: The key words are *triage acuity*; it is not a treatment area acuity.) The debate relating to this issue often surrounds established facility-specific policies for reassessment based upon the triage acuity.

A patient "acuity level" is rarely static. Patients can improve or deteriorate, and therefore an acuity level may be *updated* based upon the patient's current status. However, the acuity level assigned to the patient at the time of the triage assessment *does not change.*

REFERENCES

Agency for Healthcare Quality and Research. (2012). *Emergency severity index: A triage tool for emergency department care version 4.* Retrieved from http://www.ahrq.gov

Australasian College for Emergency Medicine. (2013a). *Guidelines on the implementation of the Australasian triage scale in emergency department (version 3).* Retrieved from https://www.acem.org.au/getattachment/d19d5ad3-e1f4-4e4f-bf83-7e09cae27d76/G24-Implementation-of-the-Australasian-Triage-Scal.aspx

Australasian College for Emergency Medicine. (2013b). *Policy on the Australasian triage scale (version 4).* Retrieved from https://www.acem.org.au/getattachment/693998d7-94be-4ca7-a0e7-3d74cc9b733f/Policy-on-the-Australasian-Triage-Scale.aspx

Buettner, J. (2013). *Fast facts for the ER nurse: Emergency room orientation in a nutshell* (2nd ed.). New York: Springer Publishing.

Gilboy, N., Tanabe, T., Travers, D., & Rosenau, A. M. (2011). *Emergency severity index (ESI): A triage tool for emergency department care, version 4. Implementation handbook 2012 edition.* AHRQ Publication No. 12-0014. Rockville, MD: Agency for Healthcare Research and Quality.

Manchester Triage Group. (2014). *Emergency triage: Manchester Triage Group* (3rd ed.). Chichester, UK: John Wiley & Sons.

Triage First, Inc. (2013). *ED triage: Comprehensive course.* Asheville, NC: Author.

9

Documentation

Rebecca S. McNair

Triage is a process, not a place. Therefore, triage entails the process of patient throughput from point-of-entry to patient disposition and transfer of care to the next provider. Documentation of this process is mandatory and serves multiple purposes. These purposes include creating an archive of the patient with the goal of ensuring quality patient care; proving adherence to professional standards of care, and organizational policies and procedures; and advocating for the patient through clear communication between care providers. Many documentation components are necessary for a comprehensive triage assessment, although some of this documentation may occur at the bedside if immediate bedding is implemented after a rapid triage assessment. (See Chapter 5 for additional information on this topic.)

Upon conclusion of this chapter, you will be able to:

1. Recognize a systematic approach for the collection and recording of necessary triage data in the patient medical record
2. State one mnemonic to guide triage documentation
3. Identify elements required for meeting best practice in triage documentation

ESSENTIAL COMPONENTS OF GOOD DOCUMENTATION

The hallmarks of good documentation include *brevity* and *clarity*. To be both brief and clear, one must use a *systematic approach* which involves performing the assessment and concordant documentation in essentially the same manner every time, using a SOAP (*Subjective, Objective, Assessment, Plan*) format. The essential components of good documentation for a comprehensive (2–5 minute) triage assessment include:

Arrival Time

- Actual time of initial patient arrival to the facility

Time Seen by the Triage Nurse

- Actual time at which rapid and comprehensive triage assessments begin (see Chapter 5 for additional information)

Documentation of Subjective Assessment of the Chief Complaint

- *Reason for visit:* Subjective narrative component of triage documentation; this is the *symptom-driven chief complaint* as ascertained by the triage nurse through questioning, observation, or both—not simply the patient's stated reason for visit
- *Medications, allergies* (agent *and* specific adverse reactions)
- *Pertinent mandatory screenings:* Organizations vary regarding mandatory screenings (e.g., fall risk, intimate partner violence, nutritional screen, etc.); thus, follow your facility protocol
- *Pain assessment:* This parameter of the patient's subjective experience *must* be noted in every visit and includes physical, psychological, and social distress

FAST FACTS in a NUTSHELL

- Patients may misinterpret their symptoms. If a patient presents with a complaint of "migraine headache," it is the triage nurse's responsibility to ask the patient what symptoms he or she is having and then document the chief complaint in symptom form, such as "headache, photophobia, and nausea." When using electronic medical records with pre-populated chief complaint fields, consider the option to provide a free text note of the chief complaint if the system does not support a symptom-driven chief complaint. Remember that it is not a nursing function to document diagnostically.
- Never document as a chief complaint by referring to an organ or structure that you cannot see (e.g., kidney pain, stomach pain, rib pain). Refer instead to the anatomical location (e.g., RUQ [*right upper quadrant*] abdominal pain).

Documentation of Objective Assessment of the Chief Complaint

- General body systems observations, including:
  - *Mode of arrival:* An ambulatory patient, mobile with use of an assistive device (e.g., cane, walker, or wheelchair), or uneven gait (e.g., staggering, limping)
  - *Abnormal observations:* Hygiene, clothing, odor resembling alcohol on breath
  - *Respiratory status:* Respiratory rate, rhythm, effort (e.g., labored or unlabored)
  - *Neurological status:* Alert and oriented to person, time, place, and event
  - *Integumentary status:* Skin color, temperature, moisture
- Pertinent vital signs
- Pain assessment (objective observations)
- Focused physical assessment pertinent to chief complaint

═══════════════════════════*FAST FACTS in a NUTSHELL*

- The necessity of obtaining an accurate weight in *kilograms* for patients presenting to the emergency department is well documented. Many medications require weight-based dosing.
- Medication errors generating from the emergency department occur with a frequency of 20.7%. Nurses and physicians who estimate patient weights only come within 10% of the patient's actual weight approximately 50% of the time (Pennsylvania Patient Safety Advisory, 2009).

Assessment Statement

- Acuity category or severity index rating based on a statistically valid and reliable triage acuity scale or severity index

Plan

- Any diagnostic tests and care ordered
- Disposition (initial disposition if the patient is assigned to wait, as well as treatment area disposition)

Interventions

- Diagnostics and care rendered (e.g., x-ray, ice, medications, etc.)

Evaluation

- Effectiveness of triage interventions initiated

Reassessments

- Should be recorded at appropriate intervals as dictated by triage acuity scale, facility, or organizational guidelines, and should reflect the standard of care for each acuity category
- Should occur if a change is noted by the patient, spouse, or nursing or ancillary staff

FAST FACTS in a NUTSHELL

- Patients interpret the word *pain* as having a very specific meaning. Try rephrasing your questions as follows: "Are you having *any discomfort* at all? Are you experiencing any unusual feelings? Can you describe those feelings?" Use the mnemonic PQRST to obtain additional information.
- Documentation of pain must include both subjective *and* objective elements. If the patient reports a high level of pain and the nurse assigns a low triage acuity category, then supportive data must be documented to validate that lower acuity level. For example:
  - Subjective: Patient states he is "in severe pain and cannot even work. Rates pain 8 on a 0 to 10 scale."
  - Objective: Patient observed laughing and walking around waiting area, talking on mobile phone.

DOCUMENTATION OF AMA, LPT, LWOT, LPMSE

See Chapter 7 for information regarding patients' leaving prior to care.

MNEMONICS TO GUIDE DOCUMENTATION

Mnemonics can help the triage nurse drive questioning, which facilitates documentation. See Chapter 28 for more information regarding mnemonics that assist in pediatric documentation.

Mnemonic: OLD CART

Onset of symptoms
Location of symptoms
Duration of symptoms

Characteristics of symptoms described by patient
Aggravating factors
Relieving factors
Treatment administered before arrival and outcome

Mnemonic for Pain Assessment: PQRST

Provokes and Palliates
- What makes it worse? What makes it better?

Quality
- What does the pain feel like (e.g., aching, sharp, dull, pressure, stabbing, etc.)?

Region and Radiation
- Where is the pain located? Does it radiate to any other part of the body?

Severity and associated Symptoms
- Use of a 0 to 10 visual analog scale: 0 = none and 10 = worst pain imaginable
- Mild–moderate–severe (severe pain significantly interferes with activities of daily living)
- Other pain rating scales
- Pediatric pain assessment scales

Timing and Temporal relations
- Onset and duration?
- Constant or intermittent pain?

═══════════════════════════════*FAST FACTS in a NUTSHELL*

- Sometimes words are documented inappropriately, most likely due to confusion regarding their meaning. Knowing the definition behind the words you use in documentation is important. Examples of words commonly confused are "lethargic," "drowsy," "irritable," and "fussy."
- "Lethargic" versus "drowsy": "Lethargy" can be defined as unusual sleepiness, denotes a significant neurological sequela, and is evidenced by a child who cannot be easily aroused. "Drowsiness" would be used for the most common symptom after crying, or from a lack of sleep, and the child can be easily aroused.

- "Irritable" versus "fussy": "Irritability" may indicate a serious neurological event. Children who are truly irritable are unable to be consoled (by a caregiver, bottle, pacifier, or other comfort measures). Such inconsolable crying is often seen in the child who presents with meningitis. "Fussy" infants and children have many reasons for crying or being fussy, including discomfort, fever, anxiety, hunger, or exhaustion (Triage First, 2012).

Websites for additional information on pain assessments include:

- www.aspmn.org/Pages/default.aspx
- www.americanpainsociety.org
- www.painedu.org/Downloads/NIPC/Pain_Assessment_Scales.pdf
- www.eperc.mcw.edu/EPERC/FastFactsIndex/ff_117.htm

REFERENCES

Pennsylvania Patient Safety Advisory. (2009). Medication errors: Significance of accurate patient weights. *Pennsylvania Patient Safety Advisory, 7*(3), 10–15. Retrieved from http://www.patientsafetyauthority.org

Triage First, Inc. (2012). *ED triage: Comprehensive course; ED triage systematics, documentation lecture.* Asheville, NC: Author.

10

Core Measures

Lynn Sayre Visser

Core measures are national initiatives used to drive quality patient care with the goal of achieving best patient outcomes. Hospitals follow core measure guidelines helping them provide exceptional care grounded by evidence-based research. Approximately 10 core measures exist with several specifically influencing emergency department (ED) care. In addition to hospital-based employees, telephone triage nurses, pre-hospital personnel, and urgent care staff should be aware of these measures so actions can be taken to ensure the patient receives appropriate care. Acute myocardial infarction (AMI), pneumonia, and stroke are the most common core measure presentations seen in the ED, with sepsis being a likely up-and-coming core measure.

Upon conclusion of this chapter, you will be able to:

1. Identify screening and assessment questions for three core measure initiatives
2. Describe three core measure treatment goals
3. List key core measure nursing actions

CORE MEASURES

Triage nurses play an important role with core measures. Meeting core measure timelines requires the triage nurse to be familiar with the associated criteria. Asking the right questions at the right time is essential. Consistently applying screening measures aids in appropriately identifying patients who are at risk for these time-sensitive diagnoses. Early recognition leads to initiation of treatment that can greatly enhance patient outcomes.

For the purposes of this book, a basic understanding of signs and symptoms of many conditions is assumed. Jennifer Buettner's *Fast Facts for the ER Nurse: Emergency Room Orientation in a Nutshell* provides more detailed signs and symptoms related to the core measure presentations discussed and can further supplement the knowledge of the triage nurse.

ACUTE MYOCARDIAL INFARCTION (AMI)

AMI can be symptomatic or asymptomatic. Early recognition is critical since mortality and morbidity rates are increased in the face of an AMI. *Remember: Time is muscle!*

Screening Questions/Assessment

Questions you will want to ask to determine the level of concern for an AMI center on the presence of the following symptoms:

- Chest pain? If the patient responds "yes" to an inquiry about the presence of chest pain, ask the PQRST (provokes and palliates; quality; region and radiation; severity and associated symptoms; timing and temporal relations) questions, including whether the pain radiates to the back, shoulder, arms, jaw, or neck.
- Associated shortness of breath or dyspnea?
- Epigastric pain, nausea, vomiting, associated sweating, or diaphoresis?
- Dizziness, syncopal episode(s), or chest pain unrelieved with rest?

Risk Factors for AMI

- *Modifiable risk factors:* Obesity, tobacco use, substance abuse, high cholesterol, elevated serum lipids, diabetes, hypertension, decreased physical activity, and psychosocial issues
- *Nonmodifiable risk factors:* Ethnicity (Caucasian at highest risk), increasing age, gender (men generally more at risk than women), genetic predisposition, and family history of heart disease

Treatment Goals

Upon suspicion of an AMI, treatment should be initiated with careful consideration to mandated time frames indicated in Table 10.1.

Utilizing a core measure order set can assist staff with meeting treatment guidelines. Most likely the triage nurse will not be the one to ensure follow through on all elements of the guidelines, but this nurse holds the key to *identifying* individuals who need the core measure treatment initiated. In some facilities, the triage nurse indicates the initiation of the core measure order set in the computer system or places a copy of the order set on the paper chart. This practice raises awareness to the care team.

You may be thinking, there is no possible way I can get an electrocardiogram (ECG) within the first 10 minutes at *my facility!* Obtaining

TABLE 10.1 Acute Myocardial Infarction Treatment Goals	
Time Frame	**Treatment**
Within 10 minutes of arrival	Electrocardiogram (ECG)
Upon arrival	Aspirin
Before giving a thrombolytic	Chest x-ray (CXR)
< 30 minutes	Thrombolytic
< 90 minutes	Percutaneous coronary intervention

the ECG at triage can be difficult due to space constraints, but the necessity of obtaining the ECG cannot be overemphasized. The ECG can occur on a gurney, in a reclining chair, or upright if there are no other options. Some locations and physical positions may be less than optimal for both the patient and staff but flexibility (literally!) may be required to initiate the preliminary ECG.

Key Nursing Actions at Triage

• Document arrival time and use this time as "time zero" for implementing care
• Initiate basic life support measures for airway, breathing, and circulation management
• Obtain the ECG within the first 10 minutes of patient arrival; refer to your facility protocol
• Initiate an ST-segment elevation myocardial infarction (STEMI) alert per protocol if applicable; a predesignated team of people come together rapidly to provide the standard of care (e.g., rapid response team, nurses, physicians, radiology, lab, pharmacy staff)
• Transport the patient from triage to the treatment team immediately by wheelchair or gurney
• Anticipate the need for oxygen, venous access, chest x-ray (CXR), medications, and laboratory testing
• Notify the provider of the high acuity patient presentation
• Flag the medical record as a time-sensitive situation to increase staff awareness

Although you may not personally perform each intervention at triage, know your policies and advocate appropriately so the patient obtains timely care. Current guidelines for cardiac care are available from the American College of Cardiology/American Heart Association and may be retrieved from http://my.americanheart.org/professional/StatementsGuidelines/ByTopic/TopicsA-C/ACCAHA-Joint-Guidelines_UCM_321694_Article.jsp

- The triage nurse plays a pivotal role in identifying individuals who potentially meet core measure criteria and ensuring that specific core measure treatment is initiated.
- Meeting the timelines with 100% efficiency not only provides quality evidence-based care and patient safety, but shows the ability of the hospital to follow requirements developed by The Joint Commission and the Centers for Medicare and Medicaid Services.

STROKE

A stroke, or cerebrovascular accident, is the interruption of cerebral blood flow. The onset of neurological symptoms within the past 48 hours is representative of an acute stroke. As in an AMI, recognition of a stroke is essential for reducing patient morbidity and mortality. Patients with evolving ischemic strokes lose 1.9 million neurons and 14 billion synapses per minute, aging the human brain by 3.6 years per hour (Saver, 2006). This translates to the destruction of 7.5 miles or 12 kilometers of myelinated fibers (Saver, 2006). Every 4 minutes an American dies of a stroke (Go et al., 2012). These alarming statistics validate the need for rapid initiation of treatment. *Remember: Time is brain tissue!*

Screening Questions/Assessment

To determine level of concern for a possible stroke, consider whether there was sudden onset of any of the following signs and symptoms:

- Presence of confusion, difficulty understanding others, or slurred speech?
- Visual disturbances in one or both eyes?
- Presence of one-sided arm, leg, or face weakness or numbness?
- Severe headache without known cause?
- Dizziness or difficulty walking or maintaining balance?
- Impaired physical coordination? (National Stroke Association, 2014)

Finally, inquire when the patient was *last seen normal* (at his or her baseline) as this information is critical and will influence the treatment plan.

Risk Factors for Stroke

- *Modifiable risk factors:* High blood pressure, diabetes, atherosclerosis, high cholesterol, atrial fibrillation, circulation problems, obesity, alcohol use, tobacco use (e.g., smoking or chewing), and physical inactivity
- *Non-modifiable risk factors:* Age, gender, race, family history, previous stroke or transient ischemic attack (TIA), and patent foramen ovale (National Stroke Association, 2014)

Treatment Goals

A patient who exhibits signs and symptoms of a stroke will need a rapid evaluation and computed tomography (CT) scan of the head to determine the type of stroke (e.g., hemorrhagic or ischemic) and candidacy for thrombolytic therapy or other interventional treatment. The actions of the triage nurse should be the same regardless of the diagnostic outcome. When the following guidelines established by National Institutes of Neurological Disorders and Stroke (NINDS) are followed, the arriving patient is given the opportunity to obtain the best possible outcome (Jauch et al., 2013). Current guidelines for stroke care are available from the American Heart Association/American Stroke Association in the Guidelines for Early Management of Patients with Acute Ischemic Stroke (Jauch et al., 2013). Table 10.2 outlines care guidelines.

Identification of stroke patients focuses on the time the patient was *last seen normal.* Patients receive the most substantial benefit from the initiation of intravenous thrombolytic therapy when given within the first hour of symptom onset, although thrombolytic therapy given up

TABLE 10.2 Stroke Care Treatment Goals

Time Frame	Treatment
0–10 minutes	Perform a triage assessment Neurological screening ED medical provider evaluation
0–15 minutes	Activate stroke team
0–25 minutes	Obtain computed tomography (CT) scan of head
0–45 minutes	Head CT interpretation
< 1 hour	Determine candidacy for fibrinolytics Door-to-drug time
3 hours from onset of symptoms	Begin post-fibrinolytic pathway

to 3 hours after the beginning of symptoms has significant benefits. The Cincinnati Prehospital Stroke Scale or the Los Angeles Prehospital Stroke Screen are tools that can be used at triage to rapidly assess a patient for stroke symptoms. Many facilities utilize the National Institutes of Health Stroke Scale (NIHSS), a valid and reliable clinical stroke assessment tool that determines the severity of the condition of the stroke patient and helps guide treatment. Use of this tool should *not delay* movement of the patient from triage to the treatment team. *Time is of the essence;* thus, quick identification of a potential stroke candidate and critical thinking skills at triage can significantly impact the patient outcome and possibly prevent a catastrophic permanent disability.

Key Nursing Actions at Triage

- Document arrival time and use this time as "time zero" for implementing care (refers to the time frames indicated in Table 10.2)
- Initiate basic life support measures for airway, breathing, and circulation management
- Begin rapid identification of stroke signs and symptoms
- Determine the time when the patient was last seen normal
- Initiate a stroke alert/stroke team activation per facility protocol
- Notify the medical provider of the high acuity patient presentation
- Flag the medical record as a time-sensitive situation to increase staff awareness

PNEUMONIA

A patient who arrives with symptoms that raise suspicion of pneumonia needs a quick screening to determine if criteria exist that require expedited treatment to meet core measure timelines. Processes should be in place to capture the right candidates. Overcrowding can lead to increased wait times and delays in treatment if devised systems are not adhered to. Timely antibiotic administration is the essential component of this core measure. *Remember: Time is multiplying organisms and increasing infection!*

Screening Questions/Assessment

When evaluating a patient for a suspicion of pneumonia, consider whether any of the following signs and symptoms are present:

- Fever, fatigue, weakness, or malaise?
- Shortness of breath, cough, or chest discomfort?
- Adventitious lung sounds?
- Vital sign abnormality, including respiratory rate > 20 breaths per minute, heart rate > 100 beats per minute (bpm), pulse oximetry < 95% on room air, or temperature > 100.4 °F (38 °C)?

Risk Factors for Pneumonia

- Cancer, chemotherapy, or other cancer treatments; recent organ transplant; human immunodeficiency virus (HIV); heart disease; chronic bronchitis or emphysema; nausea, vomiting, poor gag reflex, or difficulty swallowing; recent viral infection, cold symptoms, or upper respiratory tract infection; elderly, recent hospital stay, or living in a long-term care facility; recent chest injury or surgery; prolonged bed rest

Treatment Goals

- The goal for door-to-antibiotic time is less than 6 hours (time begins to run upon patient arrival)
- Prior to antibiotics being administered, two sets of blood cultures should be obtained
- Obtain a CXR as soon as possible after patient arrival

Key Nursing Actions at Triage

- Document arrival time and use this time as "time zero" for implementing care
- Initiate basic life support measures for airway, breathing, and circulation management
- Begin rapid identification of pneumonia signs and symptoms
- Initiate advanced triage protocols per facility policy or advocate for orders
- Notify the provider of the time-sensitive patient presentation
- Flag the medical record as a time-sensitive situation to increase staff awareness

════════════════════════ *FAST FACTS in a NUTSHELL*

Knowing core measure treatment goal timelines is an essential first step in meeting the goals! Referencing core measure order sets helps staff focus on the specific criteria and prevents missing key components.

OTHER MEASURES AND POTENTIAL UP-AND-COMING CORE MEASURES

Additional core measures including pediatric asthma and congestive heart failure exist. However, many of these other core measures do not have the same level of time sensitivity as the core measures discussed in this chapter. Please refer to www.jointcommission.org or www .qualitymeasures.ahrq.gov for additional information.

SEPSIS, SEVERE SEPSIS, AND SEPTIC SHOCK

Sepsis, severe sepsis, and septic shock are serious health concerns requiring timely, appropriate intervention. To date sepsis is not a core measure, but patient outcomes rely on time-driven care. Thus, understanding the guidelines for caring for septic patients is imperative. Additional information on this topic is available at www .survivingsepsis.org. *Remember: Time is multiplying organisms, systemic involvement, organ dysfunction, and hypoperfusion!*

Screening Questions/Assessment

Two important screening questions for sepsis exist. Each patient presenting to your facility should be screened using the three-part process below.

Part I: Infection

Is there presence or suspicion of an infection? Is the patient taking antibiotics? If "yes" to either question, continue to part II.

Part II: Systemic Inflammatory Response Syndrome (SIRS) Criteria

Determine whether the patient meets at least *two* of the criteria listed below:

- Altered mental status from the patient's baseline
- Temperature > 101.0 °F (38.3 °C) or < 96.8°F (36 °C)
- Heart rate > 90 beats per minute
- Respiratory rate > 20 breaths per minute
- White blood cell count (WBC) > 12,000 μL^{-1} or WBC count < 4000 μL^{-1}
- Hyperglycemia > 140 mg/dL? (Evaluation for Severe Sepsis Screening Tool, n.d.)

If both part I and part II are met, proceed to part III.

Part III: Acute Organ Failure

Screening for the presence of organ dysfunction criteria at triage should also occur and includes:

- Systolic blood pressure (SBP) < 90 mmHg or mean arterial pressure (MAP) < 65 mmHg
- SBP decrease > 40 mmHg from baseline

- Lactate > 2 mmol/L (18.0 mg/dL)
- Platelet count < 100,000 µL
- International normalized ratio (INR) > 1.5 or partial thromboplastin time (PTT) > 60 seconds
- Creatinine > 2.0 mg/dL
- Urine output < 0.5 mL/kg/hour for 2 hours
- Increased oxygen need to maintain oxygen saturation > 90% (Society for Critical Care Medicine, n.d.)

This information is important for the triage nurse as many facilities initiate nursing protocols at triage while the patient waits for a treatment bed. Early initiation of nursing protocols may uncover the most common signs of acute organ failure. Severe sepsis is met if *both* a suspicion of infection and the presence of organ dysfunction exist.

Risk Factors for Sepsis

- Presence of a bacterial infection anywhere in the body, including the bloodstream, bones, skin, or organs; surgical wounds, burns, or decubitus ulcers; invasive lines (e.g., central lines), surgical drains, or breathing tubes
- Immunocompromised status

Treatment Goals

To be completed within the first 3 hours from time of patient arrival:

- Obtain blood lactate level
- Draw blood cultures, preferably before initiating antibiotics
- Administer broad-spectrum antibiotics
- Administer crystalloid fluid at 30 mL/kg for a lactate level ≥ 4 mmol/L or hypotension (Dellinger et al., 2012)

Note: Treatment goals also exist for the first 6 hours of care. Refer to www.survivingsepsis.org for further information.

Key Nursing Actions at Triage

- Document arrival time and use this time as "time zero" for implementing care
- Initiate basic life support measures for airway, breathing, and circulation management
- Recognize the potential patient in severe sepsis or septic shock
- Use a severe sepsis screening tool to identify patients who meet criteria; the Surviving Sepsis Campaign offers a screening tool at www.survivingsepsis.org/SiteCollectionDocuments/ScreeningTool.pdf

- Initiate a sepsis alert per facility protocol
- Raise awareness of the patient arrival to the treatment team
- Start advanced triage protocols per policy or advocate for medical provider treatment orders

FAST FACTS in a NUTSHELL

- Be familiar with the screening criteria for a patient with a possible AMI, stroke, pneumonia, and sepsis.
- Time is heart muscle! Time is brain! Time is multiplying organisms and increasing infection! As the triage nurse, you hold the key that can be the difference between life and death. Time is of the essence!

REFERENCES

Dellinger R., Levy, M., Rhodes, A., Djillali, A., Gerlach, H., Opal, S. . . . Surviving Sepsis Campaign Guidelines Committee including the Pediatric Subgroup. (2013). Surviving sepsis campaign: International guidelines for management of severe sepsis and septic shock. *Critical Care Medicine, 41,* 580–637.

Evaluation for Severe Sepsis Screening Tool. (n.d.). Retrieved November 1, 2014, from http://www.survivingsepsis.org

Go, A. S., Mozaffarian, D., Roger, V. L., Benjamin, E. J., Berry, J. D., Borden, W. B., . . . Turner, M. B. (2012). Heart disease and stroke statistics—2013 update: A report from the American Heart Association. *Circulation,* e2–241. Retrieved March 18, 2015, from http://www.circ.ahajournals.org/content/127/1/e6

Jauch, E., Saver, J., Adams, J., Bruno, A., Connors, J., Damaerschalk, B., . . . Yonas, H. (2013). Guidelines for the early management of patients with acute ischemic stroke. *Stroke, 44,* 870–947. Retrieved March 18, 2015, from http://stroke.ahajournals.org/content/suppl/2013/01/29/STR.0b013e318284056a.DC1/Executive_Summary.pdf

National Stroke Association. (2014). *Am I at risk for a stroke?* Retrieved from http://www.stroke.org

Saver, J. (2006). Time is brain-quantified. *Journal of the American Heart Association, 37,* 263–266.

Society for Critical Care Medicine. (n.d.). Evaluation for Severe Sepsis Screening Tool. Retrieved November 1, 2014, from http://www.survivingsepsis.org

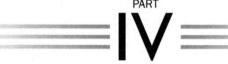

PART

IV

Current Trends Impacting Triage Nursing

11

Urgent Care Triage

Valerie Aarne Grossman

The purpose of urgent care centers (UCCs) is to serve the urgent medical needs of patients in a cost-effective, high-quality manner outside of the more expensive hospital emergency departments (EDs). The urgent care arena is not intended to care for emergent or high acuity medical needs of patients. These are different settings, managed by different groups, aimed at different populations, but all with the same end goal: to provide a health care service to those in need in an appropriate manner. This chapter begins the discussion of the growing use of UCCs, which operate under a variety of names yet all with a similar purpose.

Upon the conclusion of this chapter, you will be able to:

1. State three benefits that UCCs offer to those seeking care
2. Discuss the role of triage in a UCC
3. Understand the necessity of UCCs

BACKGROUND

UCCs began in the 1980s as a solution to the limitation of the private physician's office and the rapidly growing census of the already crowded EDs. Over the past 30 years, these centers have continued to grow in number, improve access to care, lower episodic health care costs (especially after-hours), and provide a wider variety of services than were initially available. Depending on the center, they may offer:

- Laboratory services
- Medication administration (e.g., influenza vaccines)
- Radiology services
- Care to patients across the age spectrum
- Drug testing
- Application of splints and casts (simple bone fractures)
- Simple laceration repair

- Administration of intravenous hydration
- Occupational health services
- School and employment physical exams

Many target their hours of operation to overlap peak hours of the local EDs or provide coverage when private physician offices are typically closed (e.g., weekday evenings, weekends, holidays).

There are an estimated 9,000 UCCs in the United States that care for 70 to 160 million patients annually (Urgent Care Association of America, 2011a). Over the past decades, as many hospitals (and their EDs) have closed their doors, the number of displaced patients seeking care for their urgent health needs has increased. This number is projected to grow as more people gain insurance through the Patient Protection and Affordable Care Act and seek assistance from the health care system.

STAFFING

The skill level and number of personnel working at a UCC will depend on the size and scope (facility specific), and governing agency regulations, and is tailored to the exact services offered. Staffing could include:

- Physicians
- Physician assistants
- Nurse practitioners
- Radiologic or laboratory technologists, or both
- Registered nurses
- Registration clerks
- Licensed practical/vocational nurses
- Patient care technicians (unlicensed)

REGULATIONS

There is a great variety in the regulations that a UCC may need to follow. Each professional working in the center will have his or her own licensing guidelines to follow, and the center itself will need to comply with the governing rules under which it is credentialed. For example, if the UCC is part of a hospital setting, the center will need to comply with the Emergency Medical Treatment and Active Labor Act (EMTALA).

FAST FACTS in a NUTSHELL

The regulations under which a center will operate usually depend on the "owner" of the clinic (e.g., physician owned, hospital owned, corporation owned, etc.).

The presence of UCCs continues to expand. According to the Urgent Care Association of America (2011b), more than 300 new UCCs open each year. In addition, retail medical clinics (RMCs) are being built in national pharmacy and grocery chains. In 2012, there were over 1,000 such clinics. It is estimated that more than $4 billion annually can be saved when patients utilize the services of UCCs or RMCs instead of hospital EDs (Mann, 2014). The services delivered by each UCC or RMC may vary to meet the needs of the community, the practice vision of the owner, or the licensure of those it employs. No intention of an ongoing provider–patient relationship exists, as care is delivered on an episodic basis, only.

TRIAGE

The typical UCC operates on a "first-come, first-served" basis, although when an acute or emergent patient walks in the door, he or she should be seen ahead of all waiting. In larger centers, a system of triage may be employed similar to the 5-tier triage system used in an ED. There is no "master list" of appropriate patient complaints that would be cared for at an UCC, as any complaint may have a more critical underlying component. However, typical minor complaints that could be cared for at an UCC may include:

- Rash
- Minor laceration
- Upper respiratory illness
- Dental complaints
- Minor eye complaints
- Nausea, vomiting, diarrhea
- Dysuria
- Minor trauma
- Muscle aches and pain
- Headache
- Ear pain
- Sore throat
- Sunburn
- Suture removal
- Minor skin infection
- Sprains or strains
- Medication refill
- Nosebleed
- Fever
- Foreign body removal
- Sexually transmitted infection

For specific triage applications, please refer to the "red flag" patient presentation chapters that comprise Part V.

FAST FACTS in a NUTSHELL

Any minor complaint can easily have a complicated, hidden origin. Quickly rule out serious conditions for simple complaints or triage to a higher level of care delivery.

UCCs and RMCs play an important role in the overall delivery of health care in the United States. They fill the gap between scheduled appointments in a physician's practice and the overcrowded EDs, which are utilized for any health need by a large and varied population. These alternatives offer a wide range of health care services, at a more cost-effective rate than a hospital ED, and are often open at convenient hours and locations for those seeking care.

REFERENCES

Mann, C. (2014, January 16). Centers for Medicaid and CHIP Services (CMCS) informational bulletin. Retrieved from http://www.medicaid.gov/Federal-Policy-Guidance/Downloads/CIB-01-16-14.pdf

Urgent Care Association of America (2011a). The case for urgent care [white paper]. Retrieved May 19, 2014, from http://www.ucaoa.org/docs/WhitePaperTheCaseforUrgentCare.pdf

Urgent Care Association of America (2011b). Urgent care statistics and benchmarking. Retrieved March 1, 2014, from http://www.ucaoa.org/docs/urgentcaremediakit.pdf

Electronic Medical Record Considerations

Dawn Friedly Gray

Electronic medical records (EMRs) are being introduced everywhere as a result of government regulations requiring facilities to follow meaningful use guidelines and improve patient care through increased access to electronic documentation. This chapter reviews key concepts to remember about triage EMR documentation. Documentation should accurately reflect decision-making processes and support care delivery. Avoiding charting pitfalls can improve the delivery of care. Fast and accurate documentation enhances communication, improves throughput times, and leads to better patient outcomes and higher quality care.

Upon conclusion of this chapter, you will be able to:

1. List three concepts you need to know about the EMR and effective triage practices
2. State how utilizing an EMR in triage can improve patient outcomes
3. Identify three common pitfalls of the EMR in the triage setting

BENEFITS OF THE ELECTRONIC MEDICAL RECORD

Triage is a process occurring at many different times and places. It is important to use your assessment skills to elicit information when determining the priority needs of the patient and not be distracted by the structure and functionality of the EMR. Documentation should be simple and reflect the care delivered by the triage nurse.

Chief Complaint

In some EMRs, the template is selected first, and the chief complaint is delineated within the template. In other EMRs, the chief complaint is entered first, and the template stems from the chief complaint.

Regardless of the format, the documentation should be accurate, complete, and provide enough information to drive downstream processes. Adding a *simple free text note* can quickly provide *critical information* to subsequent providers that may not be conveyed through the sole use of the EMR click boxes.

FAST FACTS in a NUTSHELL

Periodically perform a self-chart review or have one of your peers do it for you. See if your documentation supports your triage decision. It is easy to "click" and move on.

Communication

Information gathered during triage can often be integrated into tracking boards in many facilities. Know which key elements are highlighted and drive treatment protocols. Become familiar with what your institution requires to be completed in triage. Listed below are some common essential documentation pieces.

- Arrival time
- Pain level
- Chief complaint
- Suicide screening
- Mode of arrival
- Allergies
- Associated symptoms
- Acuity level

Access to Information

Looking for a paper chart can take time and lead to delays. The use of an EMR makes data more accessible and allows for multiple care providers to retrieve and document information simultaneously. Immediate access to the past medical history, including allergies and medications from prior visits, is another benefit of using an EMR when determining a triage classification. For example, a patient presenting with a head injury and a Glasgow Coma Scale score of 15 may need to be assigned a higher acuity level than initially anticipated if the EMR shows the patient is taking warfarin, clopidogrel bisulfate, or rivaroxaban. Remember, triage is a process designed to quickly assess patients' needs and direct care. Prioritize and focus on accessing parts of the EMR that will result in optimizing patient care outcomes.

In the same way that the amount of detail accessed by one click in an EMR can be a positive, it can also lead to some pitfalls. Added elements and increased options to "click" can distract the provider from focusing on critical elements needed to determine a triage classification. Pitfalls include:

- Many layers to an electronic document (e.g., additional screens open with a click, which can be overwhelming)
- Nonessential screening questions that may be present in triage documents
- Too much information and cueing that may distract attention from recognizing key patient assessment signs

═══════════════════════════════════FAST FACTS in a NUTSHELL

- Familiarize yourself with the essential pieces of information your facility requires you to document during the triage process. Provide additional information as needed to validate decision-making processes and drive downstream practices to support high-quality care.
- Remain aware of functioning within the policy limitations of your facility and scope of practice.
- Pay attention to detail when you document and be careful not to make assumptions. Do not fall into the trap of "clicking" just because it is available. Be precise!

Layout of EMR

The layout and functionality of a particular EMR can also lead to barriers in documentation. The difficulty or ease of maneuverability within the triage template can influence what is documented. If you are having difficulty accessing parts of the EMR, chances are your colleagues are as well. Communicate with your management team to make sure key elements needed for assessment are easily accessible.

Downtime and Upgrades

Technology sometimes fails, which requires backup procedures to be in place. Know what the downtime procedures are for your facility. Consider reviewing downtime processes during orientation and competency assessments. As use of the EMR increases, newer nurses will not have any experience with paper charting. Taking the time to "practice" charting on paper can minimize confusion and support ongoing high-quality care during unexpected downtimes. Patient care should continue in a smooth manner with or without the support of the EMR.

An advantage of the EMR is that upgrades can be more easily integrated into the practice setting. Know when upgrades are scheduled to occur and understand how changes may influence your practice. Be proactive in planning and continually familiarize yourself with updates in the EMR. Your patient's life may depend on it.

FAST FACTS in a NUTSHELL

- Think about how much or how little documentation is required to support the care decisions you have made.
- Make sure you document what you have observed, asked, or assessed.
- Nurses should maintain a heightened awareness during upgrades or downtime as these times may affect your ability to access patient records.
- Never let the EMR stand in the way of *looking* at the patient. Turning your back to the patient while documenting on a computer can be potentially dangerous and certainly does not deliver the customer service we should all aim to achieve. Although documentation is important, ensuring staff safety and performing a patient assessment should always come first.

13

Provider in Triage

Lynn Sayre Visser

Overcrowding in emergency departments (EDs) is a nation-wide challenge. A new focus that links hospital reimbursement to customer satisfaction adds another element to the practice of patient care. These issues have prompted creative methods of resource utilization. One solution is to place a provider (e.g. medical doctor, doctor of osteopathy, nurse practitioner, or physician assistant) in triage to mitigate overcrowding challenges, reduce wait times, and rapidly and efficiently assess, diagnose, and initiate care for patients. This chapter offers ideas related to process and teamwork initiatives, as well as communication tips, that can help improve the communication and productivity of triage teams and enhance collaboration.

Upon conclusion of this chapter, you will be able to:

1. State the purpose of placing a provider in triage
2. Discuss the importance of communication in triage
3. List three tips for a provider in triage

PURPOSE OF PLACING A PROVIDER IN TRIAGE

Placement of a provider in triage serves a multitude of functions and offers numerous potential benefits that influence quality of care. These benefits include:

- Earlier completion of the medical screening exam (MSE)
- Faster initiation of a treatment plan (e.g., diagnostic tests, pain intervention, etc.)
- Improved patient flow and decreased departmental congestion
- Faster execution of patient disposition
- Decreased left without being seen (LWBS)
- Decreased patient length of stay (LOS)
- Increased patient and staff satisfaction

Some facilities have found that implementing the provider in triage during peak hours meets many of the purposes previously identified, resulting in increased revenue from a decreased LWBS rate. Additionally, the time from the patient's arrival at the facility to the time seen by a provider is a key factor in patient satisfaction. Many studies have demonstrated a reduction in this time frame, which is often referred to as the "door-to-doctor" or "door-to-provider" time metric. When benchmarking demonstrates a positive impact of placing the provider in triage, the hours the provider is present in triage can expand, further enhancing the positive impact on patient care.

ROLES OF STAFF AT TRIAGE

If implementing a provider in triage for the first time, developing roles for each of the team players can help build the foundation for the process. Recognizing that *flexibility* is pivotal to smooth operations at triage is essential. Although guidelines should be in place for staff roles in triage, these should be merely guidelines, with each team player collaborating to complete the work and meet patient needs. Roles to consider defining include:

- Triage registered nurse: When two nurses work together, define primary and secondary triage roles (e.g., rapid triage assessment nurse and the comprehensive triage assessment nurse); see Chapter 5 for additional information
- Provider (e.g., medical doctor, nurse practitioner, physician assistant)
- Provider scribes (assist provider with documentation)
- Secretary, unlicensed personnel, or paramedic roles

  Consider identifying who will perform the following:

- Rapid triage assessment and documentation
- Comprehensive triage assessment and documentation
- Provider documentation (e.g., provider or scribes)
- Order entry
- Initiation of provider orders (e.g., give medications, draw labs, etc.)
- Documentation of patient going to and from radiology or other departments
- Follow-up on test results if patient remains in waiting room (WR)
- Reassessment if provider orders were initiated (e.g., effects of medication, etc.)
- Discharge of patients from the WR

COMMUNICATION

Communication is an integral component of teamwork and helps to meet the purpose of placing a provider in triage. Limited or absent communication in the triage area leads to duplication of procedures, missed laboratory or radiology orders, or delayed interventions, creating inefficient processes. Ultimately the purpose of implementing a provider in triage fails and patient needs are not met. Have you ever gone to medicate a patient who stated, "The nurse just gave me that pill." Or been asked by a patient, "When am I going to x-ray?" because he had waited an hour, only to realize the x-ray was never ordered? These situations can occur frequently when effective communication and efficient processes are not in place.

Communication Within the Triage Team

Crucial communication within the triage team, whether provided verbally or with visual cues, should include:

- An understanding of the treatment plan for both the provider and nurse; this can be most easily accomplished when the provider and triage nurse work together in unison while questioning and assessing the patient
- Systems that let the team know where the patient is in the process at all times (e.g., to/from radiology, laboratory samples drawn, patient medicated, etc.); for example:
  - Indicating patient location and procedures completed in the electronic medical record
  - Utilizing a color-coded flag system that indicates the patient has gone to x-ray, needs laboratory samples drawn, and so on, if using a partial paper chart

═══════════════════════════════*FAST FACTS in a NUTSHELL*

Communication between the members of the triage team is vital since communication is the core of efficiency at triage. Without effective communication, ordering of diagnostic procedures can be missed, patient charts misplaced, and orders duplicated, leading to frustration for the staff.

Communication Between the Triage Nurse and Charge Nurse/Patient Flow Coordinator

Ongoing communication between the triage nurse and charge nurse or patient flow coordinator is essential to place patients most efficiently in the most appropriate treatment location within the facility and to assist with departmental flow. Effective communication allows for a smooth transition for both the patient and caregivers involved. Have you ever arranged for a high acuity patient in triage to be taken to a room only to find the bed is now occupied by an ambulance patient who just arrived? Suggestions for enhancing communication include:

- Maintaining an updated tracking board or electronic medical record (EMR)
- Communicating via electronic equipment (e.g., cell phones, hands-free wearable devices, alpha-numeric pagers, walkie-talkies)

Communication Between Triage Staff and Other Departments

Ensure processes are in place for the triage team to communicate directly with other departments that help facilitate patient care, diagnostic testing, facility safety, and customer service. Departments that the triage area should be able to communicate directly with include:

- Laboratory
- Radiology
- Security
- Environmental services
- Trauma team
- Administration (e.g., nursing supervisor)

Suggestions for enhancing communication between these teams include:

- Computer access to visualize patient treatment needs from different departments (for facilities with EMR)
- Placement of a simple camera positioned toward the tracking board that can be viewed from other departments (for facilities where integrative EMR does not exist)
- Utilization of different-colored flags or stickers on triage paper charts to indicate patients waiting for laboratory testing, radiology, and so on

Communication Between Triage Staff and Patients or Their Support Systems

A provider in triage can expedite the time frame in which diagnostic testing begins and treatment remedies are delivered. Although this increased efficiency is beneficial to the patient and departmental flow, too much of a good thing is not always good. If several diagnostic procedures are ordered, including laboratory tests, x-rays, and medications, and these tests are initiated rapidly, one of the problems the staff may encounter is lack of communication with the patient about the plan of care. Suggestions for enhancing communication include:

- Communicating with patients that orders initiated by the provider in triage are intended to seek diagnostic answers more rapidly and expedite their ED visit
- Explaining that early initiation of tests may require the patient to move from the WR and back multiple times or require initiation of an intravenous line at a later time
- Stressing that the triage staff is doing everything possible to obtain a timely diagnosis and treatment plan and ensure the patient's medical stability
- Explaining that, if the condition warrants placement in the main ED for further treatment, additional tests may be ordered and another provider may be involved in the patient's care
- Informing the patient that he or she may need to change into a gown for further evaluation

FAST FACTS in a NUTSHELL

- In an efficient triage system, multiple staff members may interact with patients and their support systems in a short period of time. Upon the patient's arrival this initial interaction may include a parallel process involving the medical provider asking questions; the triage nurse documenting information; unlicensed personnel simultaneously obtaining vital signs, an electrocardiogram, and a weight; and registration inquiring about the spelling of the patient's name and his or her date of birth.
- Imagine how overwhelming this experience must feel to the patient. For some individuals the perception may be, "All these people are here. I must be dying!" Explain to the patient that these interactions are necessary to ensure the delivery of the highest quality of care. Let patients know the process they are experiencing is routine. The last thing a triage nurse wants is for every presenting patient to think the efficient triage process means something catastrophic is occurring.

KEY TIPS FOR THE PROVIDER

Working in triage may be uncomfortable for many providers. Historically the provider was located behind closed doors and could approach patients on his or her own time schedule.

However, in today's health care system, many providers are finding themselves one of the first faces in the patient's access to health care. A few tips for the triage provider to follow:

- Be flexible and share the space with the triage staff, registration, and so on
- Do not get caught up in the intricacies of triage and forget the little things like introducing yourself to both the patient and his or her support system; customer service *really* matters
- Determine if the provider or nurse will drive the initial patient questioning
- Work in unison with the triage team members to efficiently obtain information
- Recognize that the provider helps determine the patient destination (e.g., main ED, fast-track area, discharge from WR, etc.)
- Limit the physical exam to key assessments that are needed to determine initial orders
  - Save more lengthy assessments for the medical providers in the main ED/fast track
- When a written order for oral contrast is received from the provider while the patient is in the WR, initiate giving the contrast even if the computed tomography (CT) scan is not formally ordered at triage; this action will potentially save the patient a lot of time and prevent a situation in which the patient is left for hours on a gurney waiting for the contrast to move through the body
- Manage expectations as well as the unexpected
  - Let the patient know the provider in triage is a benefit, enabling his or her care to begin earlier while waiting for a treatment bed
  - Explain that another provider may later ask similar or additional questions and another clinical assessment may be necessary at that time
- Treat and discharge simpler cases from the triage area
  - Let patients and their family know you are doing them a service by tending to their needs quickly; in essence, your service is above and beyond what they should expect

Considerations for Triage

Open communication with the patient and support systems at triage is essential to setting the tone for expectations of the visit. Many patients arrive with chronic conditions that will most likely not be diagnosed or cured while in your facility. However, explaining that staff are excellent at ensuring no life-threatening condition exists can go a long way toward easing the worry of the people sitting in front of you. Communicate, communicate, communicate!

DISCHARGES FROM THE WR

A provider in triage can often identify simple cases that can be discharged from the WR, reserving the hot commodity of an ED bed for a higher acuity patient. The types of patients who may be treated and discharged from triage should be driven by the facility's policies and protocols. Patients to consider discharging from triage may require:

- A prescription only
- One test (e.g., x-ray, urinalysis)
- One or two treatment medications

Limiting the discharge focus to patients who need fewer resources helps maintain the flow of triage and minimizes situations in which triage personnel become bogged down with a multitude of additional tasks. The most important goals of triage must never be overlooked during the provider in triage process. All incoming patients must continually be assessed to determine how quickly they need to be seen and how sick they appear to be. In essence, a rapid triage assessment should be performed on all incoming patients. If the triage nurse becomes engulfed in initiating provider orders, rather than focusing on assessing incoming patients, the foundation of triage will be lost.

Challenges of Discharging Patients From the WR

When patients are rapidly discharged from triage, challenges can occur that include:

- Failure to complete the registration process
- Lack of education delivered to the patient about the diagnosis
- Perception on the part of the patient that not being evaluated in a room with a gurney means he or she is being "kicked to the curb" without adequate treatment

If patients are discharged from the WR, steps must be in place to ensure all elements of the patient medical record are completed in the same manner as if the patient were in a treatment bed or area. Routine discharge paperwork and explanations should be provided and not limited by overcrowding or lack of triage personnel. If corners are cut so a patient can be discharged from triage, the facility may be doing the person a disservice. Patients may not understand their discharge instructions or potential complications of their conditions, which could ultimately put them at risk.

Benefits of Discharging From the WR

When the same high level of care is delivered at triage as would be experienced in the main treatment area, discharging a patient from the triage area or WR serves many benefits. These benefits include:

- Decreased department congestion
- Decreased patient length of stay
- Increased customer satisfaction

IMPLEMENTING A PROVIDER IN TRIAGE PROGRAM

Many challenges can occur when implementing a provider in triage process for the first time. Careful planning is essential to the success of the new system. Consider the following:

- Develop a provider in triage process improvement team that includes management, registered nurses, physicians, physician assistants, nurse practitioners, unlicensed personnel, secretaries, and ancillary staff from other departments
- Identify system challenges
- Define triage team roles
- Create a plan that visually shows how the patient or staff will move within system
- Consider developing a core triage team of nurses and providers
- Trial the system for short periods of time during low census hours
- Identify what works and what does not
- Consider the impact on back-end processes and create plans for improvement
- Redefine the process
- Implement the newly defined system and identify issues
- Reanalyze the process as a team on an ongoing basis
- Implement changes as needed
- Share successes with the staff (e.g., decreased LOS and LWBS)

Even the best of systems breaks down at times. In an era of increasing patient volumes and higher acuity levels, staff should recognize that failures are an opportunity to improve. Do not give up if the first efforts at implementing a provider in triage program seem like a catastrophe. Change is hard. Change can be slow. Rather than aborting what may feel like a failed project, go back to the drawing board, reconsider goals, and try again. Your patients will benefit immensely from successful changes in the end.

- The first and foremost role of the triage nurse is to obtain a rapid assessment upon the patient's initial presentation to the facility. Assessing all incoming patients should always be the priority. Never let the efficient process of having a provider in triage interfere with the basics of the triage system unless the provider is also available to simultaneously evaluate the patient immediately upon arrival.
- System changes do not occur overnight but rather require careful planning and a team approach. Involving staff representatives from all levels of care and including staff from other departments is a must!

Advanced Triage Protocols

Dawn Friedly Gray

Increases in patient volumes and the need to expedite high-quality care have challenged health care leaders to utilize creative methods in order to meet ongoing patient demands. The use of advanced triage protocols (ATPs) is one approach to working with these challenges. This chapter reviews key concepts about ATPs and how they may be employed in your facility. Understanding the purpose of ATPs and implementing protocols during triage processes can increase patient and staff satisfaction, decrease long wait times, and improve patient throughput while simultaneously enhancing patient safety.

Upon conclusion of this chapter, you will be able to:

1. Understand what ATPs are and why they are used
2. State considerations and concerns about ATPs
3. Explain common ATPs and key points to remember

WHAT ADVANCED TRIAGE PROTOCOLS ARE AND WHY THEY ARE USED

The rate and rhythm of how patients arrive at a facility can vary greatly. Ensuring delivery of safe, high-quality care should be maintained at all times despite volume and acuity influxes. ATPs can direct care processes to continue regardless of routine or unexpected delays and are helpful when a medical provider or a treatment area is not immediately available.

Key Aspects of Protocols

- Unique to each facility and require administrative approval
  - This cannot be emphasized enough. Make sure you know the facility-specific protocols where you work!

- Based on chief complaint or specific disease conditions and the triage assessment
- Include diagnostic, therapeutic, and clinical management aspects
- Provide standardized treatment guidelines
- Evidence based

Why Use Advanced Triage Protocols?

Initiating ATPs has many benefits. Delays in care and higher lengths of stay have been shown to occur when patients seek help for lower acuity conditions. Current trends have facility administrators evaluating front-end measurements. One front-end measurement commonly assessed is the time from patient arrival to when a medical provider makes patient contact and care is initiated. This time frame is often referred to as the "door-to-doctor" or "door-to-provider" time. The implementation of ATPs can decrease wait times and expedite clinical decision making. With facility policies in place, nurses can initiate diagnostic assessments to begin immediate intervention and facilitate patient care when necessary.

Early initiation of diagnostic testing, pain management therapy, fever control treatment regimens, and tetanus vaccination protocols can decrease front-end delays and increase patient satisfaction. Timely identification of abnormal treatment results leads to safer patient outcomes and high-quality care delivery. Staff satisfaction is improved by increased nurses' autonomy and enhanced interprofessional collaboration.

FAST FACTS in a NUTSHELL

- ATPs can be used to initiate care processes and expedite patient throughput while increasing patient and staff satisfaction. Consider implementing ATPs in your facility if common delays occur.

COMMON CONSIDERATIONS AND CONCERNS

Implementation of ATPs requires careful attention to the many details and processes involved for guidelines to be successful.

Initiation of Protocols

Knowing the guidelines and expectations of your facility is imperative to appropriately initiate ATPs. For example, does your facility

policy support starting protocols on all patients or only when immediate bedding is not available? Protocols tend to be generalized according to a patient's complaint. Are you allowed to tweak ATPs if
the chief complaint does not match a specific treatment pathway? For
example, a chief complaint of abdominal pain in a 50-year-old man
with a past medical history (PMH) of alcoholism may require different testing than a 50-year-old male with abdominal pain and no PMH.
Also, initiation of protocols is only beneficial if adequate support staff
are available to perform the ordered laboratory testing and electrocardiograms (ECGs), and transport patients to radiology for x-rays,
ultrasounds, and so on.

Reviewing Results

ATPs are initiated with the hope that a treatment room and provider
will be available in a short amount of time. As we all know, this is not
always the case. There is an added responsibility on the triage nurse to
review results and identify abnormal results so they may be reported
to the medical provider. Upgrading or downgrading of the acuity level
may be necessary, which may change the care requirements for the
patient; however, the original acuity level will not change.

FAST FACTS in a NUTSHELL

- When implementing ATPs, be sure to follow guidelines from
facility policies, nurse practice acts, and governing agencies
and organizations, including the Centers for Medicaid and
Medicare Services, The Joint Commission, and the Emergency Nurses Association.
- Each nurse is responsible for knowing the limitations and
regulatory requirements governing his or her licensure.
Remain sensitive to using clinical judgment and don't hesitate to collaborate with medical providers when necessary.

Educational Requirements

Additional training is required for all nurses who initiate ATPs. Identification of unusual case presentations and quick assessment skills
are a few of the specialized skills necessary to ensure quality outcomes in patient care. Nurses need to have experience providing
care for patients of all ages with varied chief complaints to support
advanced understanding and identification of subtle and clinically
important differences in individual patient presentations. Utilizing

ATPs involves more than just picking a protocol to initiate care processes. Knowing what questions to ask to narrow down and pinpoint which protocol should be started is critical. Frequent reviews and ongoing assessments are essential to support best practices during triage processes.

FAST FACTS in a NUTSHELL

- Know what policies and guidelines govern the use of ATPs where you work. Stay abreast of evidence-based practices and encourage your facility's administration to make changes to standing protocols when indicated.
- Resist becoming complacent and following rote practices when ATPs are used.
- Your assessment skills should be patient centered and based on clinical judgment. You are the best advocate for the patient!

REVIEW OF COMMON TRIAGE PROTOCOLS

Most facilities divide ATPs into different chief complaints and patient presentations. Laboratory testing and radiology orders can vary greatly. In most states, medication administration requires a specific order and is not included in protocols. However, some facilities do include routine and time-sensitive medication administration in protocols (e.g., for acetaminophen, ibuprofen, tetanus immunization, nebulizers, aspirin, and nitroglycerin). Knowing your facility's guidelines is imperative. This section will provide general protocol categories and highlight some special considerations.

Abdominal Pain

- Complete metabolic panel (CMP) including amylase/lipase, complete blood count (CBC), urinalysis (UA), urine culture and sensitivity (urine C&S)
- Urine human chorionic gonadotropin (HCG) pregnancy test, quantitative serum HCG when appropriate
- Consider obtaining an ECG in patients older than 40 years of age; atypical presentations may be cardiac in origin
- Provide the patient with nothing by mouth (NPO)
- Additional testing (usually requires additional medical provider order) may include ultrasound (US) and computed tomography (CT)

Altered Level of Consciousness (ALOC)

- ECG
- Keep patient NPO
- Blood glucose level
- CMP, CBC, UA, and serum toxicology
- Additional testing (usually requires additional medical provider order) may include a head CT scan

Chest Pain

- ECG may be required within 10 minutes of arrival; know your facility parameters
- ST-segment elevation myocardial infarction alerts, core measure standards (see Chapter 10)
- CMP, CBC, creatinine phosphokinase (CPK), troponin; coagulation studies, including prothrombin time (PT), partial thromboplastin time (PTT), international normalized ratio (INR); chest x-ray (CXR)
- Additional testing (usually requires additional medical provider order) may include B-type natriuretic peptide (BNP), D-dimer, chest CT

Extremity Injury

- Be aware of individual facility standards and know what common views may be requested by the radiologist; x-rays can be tricky to order
- Tetanus administration is often initiated with protocols; be sure to document why/why not administered
- Consider initiation of a pain management protocol

Fever

- CMP, CBC, UA, urine C&S, blood cultures (two sets), CXR
- Consider sepsis alert; additional protocols may be included in sepsis bundles such as lactate levels and early administration of fluids and antibiotics
- Fever control protocols can be based on age, weight, or temperature and some protocols allow for alternating acetaminophen/ibuprofen administration for persistent fever in children. Don't forget to reassess temperature as indicated.

Neurological Symptoms

- CMP, CBC, PT, PTT/INR, and serum toxicology
- Blood glucose level
- CXR
- Dysphagia screening, NPO status
- Consider stroke alert as initiation of care based on timing may be critical!
- Additional testing (usually requires additional medical provider order) may include head CT scan

Pain Management

- Administration of oral analgesics can be based on age and severity
- Consider NPO status limitations and reassessment parameters

Psychological Complaints

- CMP, CBC, urine and serum toxicology
- Evaluate the need for suicide precautions

Shortness of Breath

- CMP, CBC, CPK, troponin, PT, PTT/INR, D-dimer, and BNP
- ECG and CXR
- Additional testing (usually requires additional medical provider order) may include chest CT scan

Vaginal Bleeding

- CBC and type & Rh (rhesus), urine HCG, and quantitative serum HCG if pregnant
- Additional testing (usually requires additional medical provider order) may include pelvic US

FAST FACTS in a NUTSHELL

- ATPs vary greatly and should support facility goals to improve throughput and maintain high-quality care. Consider leading a facility-based effort to implement ATPs if currently not in practice. Continually evaluate protocols to expedite care and ensure best practices.

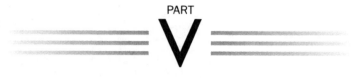

PART

V

"Red Flag" Patient Presentations

Introduction to "Red Flag" Presentations

Lynn Sayre Visser

The stage for success at triage has been set. Now what? Envision the patients rolling through the doors. How will you sort through the volumes of people presenting for medical care? Who will receive the last open gurney? Determining at triage whether a patient's complaint is a high acuity or a low acuity can be challenging. What is important to unveil is enough information to identify those conditions that are either life threatening or potentially life threatening, require time-sensitive treatment, or need rapid intervention. This chapter provides a foundation for questions, assessments, interventions, and "red flag" findings that should be considered for all patient presentations. The chapters that follow focus on the specifics of each body system.

Upon conclusion of this chapter, you will be able to:

1. State three worst-case scenarios for any patient presentation
2. List three generic triage questions that apply to all patient presentations
3. List three red flag findings for any presentation

THE TRIAGE PROCESS

Regardless of the type of facility where you work, each patient seeking medical treatment deserves the same level of diligent care that you would expect for yourself. Consistent use of best practices and a systematic approach to triage should be implemented. This systematic process involves these steps:

- Across-the-room assessment
- Eliciting the chief complaint
- The patient interview

- The physical assessment
- Vital signs

Across-the-Room Assessment

The across-the-room assessment marks the beginning of triage. To adequately assess a patient upon arrival and prevent missing critical observations, visibility of the waiting room is a must. The person performing the across-the-room assessment should use all his or her senses to obtain a general overview of the patient's physiological status. Not only is information about airway, breathing, circulation, and disability obtained through observation, but sights, sounds, and smells provide a great deal of information. This initial impression may indicate the patient is high acuity and no additional time needs to be spent obtaining information. Treatment is the priority. Remember, triage is a *process* not a place.

Eliciting the Chief Complaint

A *licensed* member of the triage team should determine the patient's chief complaint. As discussed in Chapter 9, the patient's perceived chief complaint is *not necessarily* the actual chief complaint. Thus, careful questioning by a medical person trained to obtain the chief complaint is essential.

The Patient Interview

After a clear and concise chief complaint is obtained, the triage nurse can begin to focus the questions, acquiring valuable information that helps determine the triage acuity level. To be most efficient, the triage nurse should drive the line of questioning. Asking both closed and open-ended questions is required so all pertinent information is obtained (Emergency Nurses Association, 2013).

The Physical Assessment

The triage physical assessment should be brief and driven by the chief complaint. However, the triage team must *never* become so narrowly focused that the nurse misses seeing the bigger picture. For example, if the patient has a chest complaint, investigation of both the cardiac and pulmonary systems is important and may require auscultating heart tones or lung sounds. A *visual assessment* of the area of injury or complaint is a vital component of the triage process. Patients might minimize their symptoms or not be aware of the severity of their condition. The subtle clues that become apparent during the nurse's line of questioning and physical assessment are often the answers needed to justify the acuity level. The patient may arrive complaining of a "cut to the arm" with a bandage in place. Initially, the nurse could think this is a low acuity patient, but upon removing the bandage an arterial bleed becomes evident.

Vital Signs

The degree to which vital signs are obtained at triage depends on the *urgency* of the patient's medical condition. If the across-the-room assessment provides enough information to determine a high acuity presentation and immediate bedding criteria are met, the patient goes straight to a treatment bed *without* obtaining vital signs. Vital signs are a piece of the puzzle in triage decision making and *may* lead the nurse to increase the patient acuity level.

══════════════════════*FAST FACTS in a NUTSHELL*

- The vital signs obtained upon the patient arrival serve as a baseline. Ensuring the *accuracy* of the initial set of vital signs is critical in evaluating the patient and guiding the treatment plan.
- Automatic vital sign machines should *never* be a substitute for correlating data by palpating pulses, counting the respiratory rate, and manually confirming an abnormal blood pressure. If a pulse oximetry reading is low, the nurse should consider whether the patient presentation confirms the low reading.
- Staff should always consider whether the patient has a temperature (e.g., oral, tympanic) that correlates with the skin temperature. For example, if the patient is flushed and the face is hot to touch after obtaining a temperature within normal limits, *then* the nurse should consider repeating the temperature or utilizing an alternative method.

The Patient Acuity Level

The chapters that follow will not indicate the acuity level of each presentation as many variables play a role in this decision making. Patient presentations vary, and risk factors differ. What is important to note is that the presentations discussed are worst-case scenarios that the nurse should *consider*. When the worst-case scenario cannot be ruled out, the triage nurse will likely find the presentation to be a high acuity level based on the acuity scale criteria.

WORST-CASE SCENARIOS

Under this heading in the chapters that follow, many worst-case scenarios for the specific body system are listed. The compact size of this book does not allow for every potential patient presentation or worst-case scenario to be discussed. However, the worst-case scenarios covered provide a foundation upon which the triage nurse can build. *A significant impairment to the patient's airway, breathing, circulation, or neurological status is a worst-case scenario to consider for any body system.* This point will not be repeated in each chapter but is always concerning and a clinical finding that requires action.

ESSENTIAL TRIAGE QUESTIONS, ASSESSMENT, AND INTERVENTIONS

The generic questions, assessment, and interventions that follow should be *considered* for *all* patient presentations.

Generic Questions

- Reason for your visit?
- Onset and course of symptoms?
- Recent fever?
- Recent travel (e.g., another country or region)?
- Recent exposure to an infectious disease?
- Treatment prior to arrival (e.g., medication given, ice, splint etc.)?
- Did the pain begin before the onset of symptoms?
- Pain characteristics (PQRST: provokes and palliates; quality; region and radiation; severity and associated symptoms; timing and temporal relations)?
- Associated systemic symptoms (e.g., nausea, shortness of breath, diaphoresis, feeling faint)?
- Medical, surgical, social, and family histories?
- Medications and allergies?
- Immunizations?

Generic Assessment

- *Airway:* Patent or impaired (e.g., stridor, hoarseness, drooling, facial or oropharyngeal edema)
- *Breathing:* Unlabored or labored (e.g., accessory muscle use, retractions, nasal flaring)
- *Circulation:* Skin color (e.g., pallor, cyanosis) and moisture (e.g., dry, moist, diaphoretic); pulse rate (e.g. fast or slow) and rhythm (e.g., regular or irregular); obvious bleeding

- *Disability (neurological status):* Level of consciousness including Glasgow Coma Scale (GCS) or alert, verbal, pain, unresponsive (AVPU); assessing for muscle strength in upper extremities (e.g., pronator drift, grips) and lower extremities (e.g., can the patient lift both legs?)
- Vital signs (heart rate, respiratory rate, blood pressure, pulse oximetry, and pain scale)

Generic Interventions

- Intervene immediately in patients with any airway, breathing, circulation, or disability impairment
- Consider the administration of oxygen per protocol or advocate accordingly
- Document arrival time and use this as "time zero" for implementing care; think core measure criteria and refer to Chapter 10 to initiate care if criteria are met (e.g., acute myocardial infarction, stroke, pneumonia)
- Consider the need to take action in patients with abnormal vital signs
- Give nothing by mouth (NPO) if anticipating surgical intervention or conscious sedation (e.g., suspected fracture, dislocation, etc.)
- Advocate for rapid room placement; see Chapter 5 for more on immediate bedding criteria
- Advocate for a timely diagnostic workup and initiation of care for patients with a suspicion of a high acuity presentation
- Consider transporting the patient to the treatment area by wheelchair or gurney
- Consider analgesics per protocol or advocate as needed
- Frequent patient reassessment per acuity scale criteria and facility protocols

SPECIFIC CONDITIONS

In the red flag patient presentation chapters that follow, the specific conditions listed under this heading have other questions or assessments that may lead the nurse to rule in or rule out the potential worst-case scenario. The triage nurse *will not diagnose* the patient; rather, the information obtained helps drive the questioning and may further validate the need for assigning a high acuity level. The information under each potential worst-case scenario is not intended to be comprehensive in nature but rather provides the triage nurse with key considerations while working through the nursing process.

RED FLAG FINDINGS

Each chapter presents red flag findings that aside from rare circumstances are most likely high acuity presentations. These presentations should cause the nurse to think: *Act fast!* The red flag findings that follow may be evident with any body system complaint. Additionally, the triage nurse should consider whether the patient is progressively worsening over time and use that information in conjunction with the clinical findings.

- Apneic
- Airway compromise
- Respiratory failure or distress
- Cyanotic, gray, unusually pale, diaphoretic
- Unresponsive
- Unable to speak (abnormal for patient)
- New-onset confusion
- Syncopal episode with unknown etiology
- Cardiopulmonary arrest
- New-onset limb weakness or paralysis
- Hypothermia
- Hyperthermia

FAST FACTS in a NUTSHELL

Each patient presenting to triage deserves a *nonjudgmental* assessment based on assimilation of information, including the triage interview, physical assessment, and vital signs. The triage team must *look* at the areas of complaint and consider whether all the information, including the patient's complaint, color, demeanor, and vital signs, makes clinical sense? If the answer is "no," further investigation should occur.

REFERENCE

Emergency Nurses Association. (2013). *Sheehy's manual of emergency care* (7th ed.). St. Louis, MO: Mosby.

Respiratory Emergencies

Polly Gerber Zimmermann and Lynn Sayre Visser

Determining at triage whether a complaint is respiratory or cardiac in origin can be challenging, and more often than not, the answer may not come until after diagnostic testing. Since chest pain and shortness of breath often go hand in hand, a careful review of both the respiratory and cardiac emergency chapters can help prepare the nurse for assessing these patient populations. This chapter provides a foundation for potential high acuity respiratory presentations that the triage nurse may encounter. See Chapter 17 for other presentations not addressed in this chapter.

Upon conclusion of this chapter, you will be able to:

1. State three respiratory presentation worst-case scenarios
2. List three triage questions related to a respiratory emergency
3. List three "red flag" findings of respiratory emergencies

WORST-CASE SCENARIOS

Foreign body obstruction, anaphylaxis, inhalation injury, peritonsillar abscess, epiglottitis, Ludwig's angina, tuberculosis, pneumonia, pertussis, respiratory distress or respiratory failure (e.g., asthma, congestive heart failure, chronic obstructive pulmonary disease, pulmonary edema), pulmonary embolism, tension pneumothorax).

ESSENTIAL TRIAGE QUESTIONS, ASSESSMENT, AND INTERVENTIONS

Chapter 15 is a crucial foundation for the content that follows.

Generic Questions

- Shortness of breath?
- Recent travel (e.g., concern for severe acute respiratory syndrome [SARS] or other diseases)?
- Chest pain or pain with inspiration?
- Known exposure to infectious disease?
- What began first, the shortness of breath or chest pain (if both present)?
- Recent fever?
- Presence of a cough (productive or nonproductive)?
- Recent upper respiratory infection?
- Producing sputum (e.g., color, evidence of blood, consistency)?
- Difficulty swallowing?
- Smoking history?

Generic Assessment

- Respiratory rate, depth, rhythm
- Labored or unlabored respirations
- Accessory muscle use, retractions, nasal flaring
- Number of words patient is able to speak
- Facial or oropharyngeal edema
- Drooling
- Skin color
- Level of consciousness (e.g., restlessness)
- Peripheral edema
- Lung sounds

Generic Interventions

- Initiate basic life support measures
- Institute continuous monitoring of airway for progressive airway compromise
- Place a surgical mask on the patient if cough present
- Initiate respiratory isolation if indicated
- Consider initiation of oxygen per protocol or advocate accordingly

- Respiratory complaints can progress rapidly, leading to a sudden change of acuity.
- If a patient who is waiting states that breathing is becoming more difficult, the tongue feels swollen, or he or she expresses a sense of impending doom, *believe the patient* and reassess! Triage nurses should never let their guard down since commonly this is when a patient deteriorates and adverse outcomes occur.

SPECIFIC CONDITIONS

The questions, assessment, and interventions that follow are *not* intended to be comprehensive in nature but will help guide the triage nurse through the nursing process.

Foreign Body Obstruction: Partial or Complete

1. *Questions:* Evidence of choking?
2. *Assessment:* Look for the universal choking sign (patient holding the throat and appearing anxious); difficulty or inability to speak; stridor; presence of a cough (cough may indicate partial but not complete obstruction); look of fear/impending doom; cyanosis
3. *Interventions:* Initiate basic life support protocols for foreign body removal; limit any exertion the patient puts forth

Anaphylaxis

1. *Questions:* Exposure to known or new allergen (e.g., seafood, peanuts and other nuts, insect bite or sting, iodine, latex, medication, or eggs); how many times did the exposure occur (for insect bites or stings)?
2. *Assessment:* Wheezing; rash with systemic involvement (e.g., low blood pressure); facial, tongue, or lip swelling; significant pruritus
3. *Intervention:* Anticipate medication orders (e.g., epinephrine, bronchodilators, antihistamines, steroids, H_2 blockers, and nebulizer treatments)

Inhalation Injury

1. *Questions:* What was the exposure (e.g., smoke, chemicals); how long was the exposure?
2. *Assessment:* Presence of hoarse voice; stridor or cough; black-tinged sputum; soot around nostrils; singed nasal hairs or eyebrows; mouth burns; skin color (cherry red skin is often indicative of carbon monoxide poisoning; may be more difficult to see in dark-skinned individuals)
3. *Intervention:* Anticipate the delivery of 100% humidified oxygen rapidly

FAST FACTS in a NUTSHELL

- Any evidence of an inhalation injury should be enough for the triage nurse to be highly concerned. The patient should be immediately placed in a treatment bed and the medical provider notified due to the high risk for worsening edema and airway obstruction.
- Although the patient may have a pulse oximetry reading of 100%, the triage nurse should not let his or her guard down! Carbon monoxide binding to hemoglobin gives a false high pulse oximetry reading.

Peritonsillar Abscess

1. *Questions:* Recent pharyngitis or tonsillitis?
2. *Assessment:* Unilateral tonsil swelling; unilateral neck swelling; muffled voice; older child, adolescent, or young adult; trismus (difficulty opening mouth); uvula displaced away from the area of swelling
3. *Intervention:* Anticipate the need for needle aspiration of abscess and antibiotics

Epiglottitis

1. *Questions:* Sudden onset of symptoms; sore throat (noted in 95% of patients); odynophagia or dysphagia (noted in 95% of patients)?
2. *Assessment:* Muffled voice; inspiratory stridor (a late finding); tripod position; drooling; irritability; toxic appearance
3. *Interventions:* Limit activity and stimulation during and after assessment; keep child with parent or caregiver and minimize stressors; place in position of comfort

Ludwig's Angina

1. *Questions:* Recent dental infection, tooth abscess, or mouth injury?
2. *Assessment:* Swelling of floor of mouth; elevated tongue or neck swelling; drooling
3. *Intervention:* Continuous airway monitoring

Tuberculosis

1. *Questions:* Recent fatigue, fever, chills, or night sweats; cough lasting several weeks; bloody sputum; recent weight loss; recent travel, incarceration, or exposure to a person with known tuberculosis?
2. *Assessment:* Refer to Generic Assessment, earlier
3. *Interventions:* Place a surgical mask on the patient; initiate airborne precautions (e.g., negative pressure room); communicate with other personnel per policy regarding isolation status

═══════════════════════════════*FAST FACTS in a NUTSHELL*

- One role of the triage nurse is to limit the spread of infections to staff, patients, and visitors. During flu season and when patients or visitors are coughing, masks and tissues should be handed out judiciously to reduce the spread of germs. The more frequently masks are distributed, the less uncomfortable individuals wearing them will feel.
- If in doubt about the seriousness of a potentially communicable respiratory disease, *isolate, isolate, isolate!*

Pneumonia

1. *Questions:* Fever, shortness of breath, cough, or chest discomfort; fatigue, weakness, vomiting, or malaise; prolonged bed rest or recent surgery?
2. *Assessment:* Adventitious lung sounds; vital sign abnormality
3. *Interventions:* Anticipate the need for laboratory tests (e.g., complete blood count, blood cultures), chest x-ray (CXR), and antibiotics within 6 hours of arrival to facility; see Chapter 10 for additional information on pneumonia and screening for the possibility of sepsis

Pertussis (Whooping Cough)

1. *Questions:* Severe cough (whooping sound), runny nose, fever, vomiting, or fatigue; any episodes of not breathing (apnea is noted in 67% of infants with pertussis); seizure-like activity; decreased urination or frequency of wetting diapers (Centers for Disease Control and Prevention, 2014)?

2. *Assessment:* Auscultate lung sounds; assess for signs of dehydration (e.g., absence of tearing, dry tongue/mucous membranes, and poor skin turgor)
3. *Intervention:* Initiate respiratory isolation per protocol

Respiratory Distress/Respiratory Failure

1. *Questions:* Sudden onset of symptoms; shortness of breath or chest pain; how long have you been experiencing these symptoms?
2. *Assessment:* Stridor, drooling, oropharyngeal edema; difficulty or inability to speak; skin color (e.g., pale or cyanotic); level of restlessness
3. *Interventions:* Initiate basic life support protocols; limit level of patient exertion

Pulmonary Embolism

1. *Questions:* Sudden onset pleuritic chest pain; hemoptysis; birth control pills; recent surgery; any recent relative immobility (e.g., bedridden, recent travel, or recent hospitalization); pregnancy or postpartum; history of deep vein thrombosis, pulmonary embolism, or large bone fracture (also a risk for fat emboli); current or past history of cancer?
2. *Assessment:* Unilateral leg swelling after prolonged immobility; vital signs often reveal tachycardia, tachypnea, and low pulse oximetry; restlessness; nonspecific symptoms (often the case with pulmonary embolism and may mimic other conditions)
3. *Interventions:* Consider oxygen per protocol or advocate accordingly; consider rapid need for anticoagulants (e.g., thrombolytic agents) if hemodynamically unstable

FAST FACTS in a NUTSHELL

- The classic triad of symptoms for pulmonary embolism includes sudden-onset, sharp, pleuritic chest pain (66% present with), dyspnea, and hemoptysis. All three are present only about 20% of the time. Most pulmonary emboli come from venous thromboembolism.
- At least one of the following risk factors is present in 90% of patients with a pulmonary embolism: immobility, heart disease, cancer, oral contraceptive pill use, pregnancy, previous deep venous thrombosis or pulmonary embolism, history of clotting disorders, recent surgery, hospitalization, travel, or hypercoagulability.

Tension Pneumothorax

1. *Questions:* Sudden-onset, pleuritic chest pain; severe shortness of breath; dyspnea; blunt or penetrating trauma?
2. *Assessment:* Signs of decreasing cardiac output (e.g., hypotension, tachycardia, clammy skin, ECG changes); jugular vein distention; deviated trachea (points toward the "good lung"); decreased lung sounds on auscultation; restlessness or anxiety; muffled heart sounds
3. *Intervention:* Anticipate the need for immediate needle decompression if severe hemodynamic compromise is present (do not delay treatment for a CXR)

RED FLAG FINDINGS

- Unresponsive
- Confusion or restlessness
- Speaks only 1 to 2 words or clipped sentences
- Unilateral or absent breath sounds
- Severe respiratory distress or respiratory failure
- Accessory muscle use, retractions, or nasal flaring
- Shortness of breath with associated chest pain
- Blunt or penetrating trauma to the chest
- Look of fear or describing a feeling of impending doom

REFERENCE

Centers for Disease Control and Prevention. (2014). Pertussis (whooping cough). Retrieved March 16, 2015, from http://www.cdc.gov/pertussis/about/diagnosis-treatment.html

Cardiac Emergencies

Polly Gerber Zimmermann

Chest pain can originate from many sources and may range from myocardial infarction to benign costochondritis. The key responsibility at triage is to consider the worst-case scenario in determining proper priorities. In cardiac conditions, time is muscle. Therefore, rapid intervention for suspicious cardiac conditions is imperative. This chapter provides a foundation for potential high acuity cardiac presentations that the triage nurse may encounter. See Chapter 10 for a further understanding of timelines related to electrocardiograms (ECGs), thrombolytic therapy, and percutaneous coronary intervention.

Upon conclusion of this chapter, you will be able to:

1. State three cardiac presentation worst-case scenarios
2. List three triage questions related to a cardiac emergency
3. List three "red flag" findings of cardiac emergencies

WORST-CASE SCENARIOS

Cardiac arrest, life-threatening arrhythmia, acute coronary syndrome, acute aortic dissection, pericarditis, endocarditis, tension pneumothorax, pericardial tamponade

ESSENTIAL TRIAGE QUESTIONS, ASSESSMENT, AND INTERVENTIONS

Chapter 15 is a crucial foundation for the content that follows.

Generic Questions

- Chest pain or pain with inspiration?
- Syncopal episode?
- Shortness of breath?

- What began first, the chest pain or shortness of breath (if both present)?
- Sudden onset of bilateral ankle edema?
- Associated systemic symptoms (e.g., nausea, shortness of breath, diaphoresis, feeling faint)?
- Rash? (Rule out herpes zoster)
- Recent trauma?
- History of recent upper respiratory infection (costochondritis)?
- Patient's perception of effort required to maintain oxygenation?
- Past history of similar symptoms; how is this different than previous chest pain?
- Heart disease, smoking, high blood pressure, high cholesterol, diabetes, or obesity?

FAST FACTS in a NUTSHELL

A patient with a recent history of forceful emesis, chest pain, and subcutaneous emphysema should raise suspicion in the triage nurse of the need rule out Boerhaave's syndrome (i.e., tear in the esophagus).

Generic Assessment

- Respiratory rate and characteristics (normal respiration is easy and quiet)
- Ability to speak sentences, phrases, or limited number of words between breaths
- Auscultate lung sounds
- Trachea (midline or deviated)
- Altered circulation: pale or cyanotic; delayed capillary refill
- Level of consciousness (e.g., new onset restlessness or confusion which can indicate early signs of hypoxia)
- Musculoskeletal pain (usually localized, sharp, reproducible; movement makes it worse)
- Pulse oximetry (should be 95%–100% in a healthy adult; concern is warranted if < 93% without chronic illness)

Generic Interventions

- Anticipate the need for ECG within 10 minutes of arrival and continuous monitoring
- Consider the need for oxygen for concerning chest pain, shortness of breath, or low oxygen saturation levels

The questions, assessment, and interventions that follow are *not* intended to be comprehensive in nature but will help guide the triage nurse through the nursing process.

Acute Coronary Syndrome (ACS)

1. *Questions:* Discomfort of burning, pressure, dull ache, or tightness (rather than pain) to chest, jaw, neck, epigastrium, arm, or back; symptoms with exertion but relieved by rest; pain severe enough to awaken from sleep; history of hypertension, diabetes mellitus, smoking, family history of ACS, or hypercholesteremia; previous cardiac disease, coronary interventions, pacemaker, or implantable cardioverter defibrillator (ICD); recent use of medications for erectile dysfunction (these patients should not receive nitroglycerin); recent or past use of recreational drug use such as cocaine (can cause coronary vasospasms and accelerate coronary artery disease)?
2. *Assessment:* Altered circulation: Pale, diaphoretic, cyanotic, delayed capillary refill
3. *Interventions:* Obtain an ECG within 10 minutes (refer to your facility protocol); anticipate the need for non–enteric-coated aspirin per protocol; anticipate orders for stat oxygen, ECG, intravenous access, chest x-ray (CXR), medications, and lab work

═══════════════════════════════*FAST FACTS in a NUTSHELL*

- Up to 50% of patients with ACS may not have any known risk factors. ACS is classified into unstable angina, non–ST-segment elevation myocardial infarction (MI), or ST-segment elevation MI. Signs or symptoms of cardiac ischemia, resulting in a change in the cardiac output and perfusion, or inadequate oxygenation is a concern. *Time is muscle!* After 20 minutes of ischemia, injury begins, and within 6 to 8 hours, infarction (death) begins.

- Initial negative results for ECG or cardiac enzymes are *not* definitive. Positive results for enzymes or ECG changes are typically not seen until infarction (not ischemia) occurs. Up to 6.4% of all patients with an acute MI had one normal ECG.

- Relief by nitroglycerin or "GI cocktail" is *not* legitimate as a diagnostic measure.
- Reproducible pain with pressure (classic in costochondritis) is *not* an absolute diagnostic measure. Up to 7% of patients with acute MI or unstable angina have their pain partially or fully reproduced on chest wall palpation.

Acute Aortic Dissection: Thoracic or Abdominal

1. *Questions:* Positional pain (usually not positional and the duration of pain lasts only hours); discomfort reveals ripping, tearing, abrupt pain, excruciating pain radiating to the anterior chest, back, abdomen, and/or lower extremities; history of hypertension, peripheral vascular disease, Marfan syndrome, or age $\geq$ 40 years?
2. *Assessment:* Check for significant differences in blood pressure and pulses between upper extremities; neurological deficits (e.g., paresthesia); auscultate for a heart murmur
3. *Interventions:* Consider oxygen per protocol; CXR stat to look for widened mediastinum

FAST FACTS in a NUTSHELL

- Discoloration of extremities due to poor perfusion can be indicative of aortic dissection.
- Patients with collagen vascular disorders such as Marfan syndrome are at a high risk for aortic aneurysm or dissection, or both.

Pericarditis

1. *Questions:* Sharp, sudden pleuritic chest pain that improves in upright, forward-leaning position; recent history of viral symptoms?
2. *Assessment:* Listen for pericardial rub (present in up to 69%)
3. *Interventions:* Anticipate the need for an ECG (up to 94% have abnormalities)

Endocarditis

1. *Questions:* Chest pain; joint or muscle aches; chills, fatigue, or fever; exertional shortness of breath; history of rheumatic fever or endocarditis; congenital heart abnormalities; mechanical heart valve; recent dental surgery; intravenous drug use?

2. *Assessment:* Fever; sweating; swelling of feet, legs, and/or abdomen; heart murmur
3. *Interventions:* Anticipate the need for an ECG, lab work, including two sets of blood cultures, echocardiogram, and antibiotics

Pericardial Tamponade

1. *Questions:* Sharp, stabbing pain often radiating to the shoulder, neck, back, and/or abdomen; pain worsened by deep breathing or coughing; recent open heart surgery?
2. *Assessment:* Muffled heart sounds; jugular vein distention; hypotension or signs of shock
3. *Interventions:* Anticipate the need for immediate pericardiocentesis

RED FLAG FINDINGS

- Life-threatening arrhythmia
- Sudden-onset, severe chest pain
- Blunt or penetrating trauma to the chest
- Tracheal deviation
- Cocaine or crack use with chest pain
- Patient appears uncomfortable, pale, diaphoretic, clammy, cyanotic, and/or acutely ill
- Syncopal episode associated with chest pain or shortness of breath
- Change in level of consciousness (e.g., confusion, lethargy, or restlessness)
- Angina different from the patient's usual characteristics
- Repetitive shocks by an ICD or more than three shocks in a 24-hour period
- Look of fear or feeling of impending doom

Neurological Emergencies

Reneé Semonin Holleran

There are many causes of loss of neurological function. Failure to identify concerning neurological symptoms at triage can lead to long-term disability in devastating conditions such as stroke. The history surrounding the onset of symptoms plays an important role in the care of the patient. This chapter provides a foundation for potential high-acuity neurological presentations that the triage nurse may encounter.

Upon conclusion of this chapter, you will be able to:

1. State three neurological presentation worst-case scenarios
2. List three triage questions related to a neurological emergency
3. List three "red flag" findings of neurological emergencies

WORST-CASE SCENARIOS

Stroke, seizure, Guillain-Barré syndrome, meningitis, encephalitis

ESSENTIAL TRIAGE QUESTIONS, ASSESSMENT, AND INTERVENTIONS

Chapter 15 is a crucial foundation for the content that follows.

Generic Questions

- Onset (time) of symptoms or injury (e.g., sudden or gradual)?
- Any injury associated with the onset of symptoms (e.g., fall before or after symptoms)?
- Pain characteristics; did the pain precede the symptoms (e.g., a severe headache before loss of function of an extremity or muscle weakness)?
- Presence of a fever or hypothermia?

- Past medical history including diabetes (neurological changes may be related to hypoglycemia), hypertension, injuries, medications, and vaccination history?

Generic Assessment

- Characteristics of symptoms
  - Loss of function of an extremity or the face
  - Numbness or tingling in an extremity or the face
- Presence of a fever or hypothermia

Generic Interventions

- Document arrival time and use this time as "time zero" for implementing care (stroke)
- Check glucose per protocol (determine if hypoglycemia is contributing to the neurological symptoms)
- Check ECG per protocol (atrial fibrillation maybe the cause of stroke)

FAST FACTS in a NUTSHELL

> When a patient presents with a stroke or neurological changes, knowing the exact time the patient was *last seen normal* is important for their treatment.

SPECIFIC CONDITIONS

The questions, assessment, and interventions that follow are *not* intended to be comprehensive in nature but will help guide the triage nurse through the nursing process.

Stroke

1. *Questions:* Onset of symptoms (*exact time*); have symptoms improved or worsened; dizziness or headache; any risk factors for stroke (e.g., hypertension, atrial fibrillation); history of trauma (e.g., a fall); recent or current use of anticoagulation medication?
2. *Assessment:* Assess stroke symptoms using a prehospital stroke assessment scale (e.g., Cincinnati Stroke Scale); presence of facial droop, arm drift, or slurred speech
3. *Interventions:* Determine the onset of patient symptoms (administration of tissue plasminogen activator (r-tPA) needs to occur

within 3 hours of the onset of symptoms in an ischemic stroke for best outcomes); facilitate immediate medical treatment (e.g., emergency department)

Seizures

1. *Questions:* History of seizures, tongue biting, or incontinence; what type of seizures (e.g., partial or generalized); medical history such as diabetes (hypoglycemia is potentially the cause of the seizure); postictal state; medications taken for seizures (ascertain if the patient is compliant); intentional or accidental overdose of medication; history of recent trauma or trauma due to the seizure; exposure to any toxins?
2. *Assessment:* Altered mental status; abnormal limb movement; absence of movement
3. *Interventions:* If the patient is actively seizing, place in rescue position with cervical spine precautions if a history of trauma; monitor airway and breathing; reposition airway as needed to remove obstruction; apply oxygen by mask if needed

═══FAST FACTS in a NUTSHELL

- Question the patient about a history of coronary artery disease or sudden cardiac death when assessing for seizures.
- Not all tonic/clonic activity is a "seizure"; you must also consider a dysrhythmia or syncope.

Guillain-Barré Syndrome

1. *Questions:* Any history of recent upper respiratory infection; recent vaccination; any prickling, tingling sensation, or weakness in lower extremities spreading upward; ascending paralysis; difficulty walking or inability to walk; difficulty swallowing or respiratory difficulties (late finding)?
2. *Assessment:* Muscle weakness; abnormal breathing patterns (late finding)
3. *Intervention:* Manage abnormal breathing patterns

Meningitis/Encephalitis

1. *Questions:* Severe headache; when did it start; presence of fever or recent illness, vomiting, stiff neck, generalized weakness, or an abnormal rash noticed by patient or family?

2. *Assessment:* Change in level of consciousness (e.g., confusion); focal neurological signs; muscle weakness; fever and chills; presence of purpura or petechiae (nonblanching); nuchal rigidity

3. *Interventions:* If infection is suspected, masks and gloves should be donned before performing patient care; isolate the patient per protocol as soon as possible

FAST FACTS in a NUTSHELL

- Infants with meningitis may have a high-pitched meningeal cry and are inconsolable. Be alert to decreased level of consciousness, poor feeding, vomiting, and/or bulging fontanelle.
- A neonate seizure can be overlooked due to its subtle symptoms (e.g., repetitive lip smacking, horizontal eye deviation, eyelid fluttering, pedaling, or swimming motions). *Don't be fooled!*

RED FLAG FINDINGS

- Inability to protect the airway
- Difficulty breathing
- Change in mental status from baseline
- Any neurological deficits (e.g., facial droop, loss of limb function)
- Worst headache of patient's life
- New-onset seizure
- Fever with neck stiffness
- Fever with the presence of a rash (e.g., suspicion of meningitis)

Abdominal Emergencies

Polly Gerber Zimmermann

The abdomen contains many organs, both solid and hollow, that can manifest a wide range of possible abnormal findings. Utilizing key questions helps differentiate the patient with "gas" from one with a life-threatening perforation. When triaging patients, it is important to consider the worst-case scenarios and to identify not only patients who are obviously seriously ill but also those who might be. This chapter provides a foundation for potential high acuity abdominal presentations that the triage nurse may encounter. See Chapter 20 for other presentations not addressed in this chapter.

Upon conclusion of this chapter, you will be able to:

1. State three abdominal presentation worst-case scenarios
2. List three triage questions related to an abdominal emergency
3. List three "red flag" findings of abdominal emergencies

WORST-CASE SCENARIOS

Cholelithiasis or cholecystitis, pancreatitis, peptic ulcer disease, small bowel obstruction, large bowel obstruction, incarcerated hernia, abdominal aortic aneurysm, appendicitis, diverticulitis, testicular torsion

ESSENTIAL TRIAGE QUESTIONS, ASSESSMENT, AND INTERVENTIONS

Chapter 15 is a crucial foundation for the content that follows.

Generic Questions

- Time of onset (acute versus gradual)?
- Vomiting (often seen in infectious processes)?

- Frequency and characteristics (e.g., color, food contents, bile appearance, etc.) of vomiting?
- Emesis related to pain?
  - Pain preceding vomiting suggests a potential surgical abdomen, whereas vomiting before pain is more typical of a nonsurgical condition
  - Nausea and vomiting occurring simultaneously with the onset of pain is associated with torsion, ectopic pregnancy, ureteral colic, or bowel obstruction
  - Epigastric pain relieved by vomiting is more likely to be caused by an intragastric problem
- Last bowel movement (BM)?
  - Frequency of BMs, characteristics, and normal patterns for patient?
  - Presence of dark tarry or bloody stool?
  - Guidelines for "frequent" diarrhea includes every 30 to 60 minutes for more than 6 hours, five or more episodes in the previous 24 hours, or diarrhea daily for more than 5 days
- Passing flatus?
- Recent travel (e.g., different country or region)?
- Urine frequency (especially with children or elderly who are more prone to dehydration) and characteristics (e.g., color, odor)?
- First day of last menstrual period (if premenopausal)?
- Pain worse with movement?
- Positional pain?
  - Patient often appears rigid when flat and if ambulating walks gingerly to avoid moving peritoneal area; this is often referred to as the "pelvic inflammatory disease (PID) shuffle"
- Previous history of the same or similar condition; does this feel the same as it did before?
- Lower chest trauma? (Remember: The liver and spleen are protected by the lower rib cage but still vulnerable to injury)
- Recent hospitalization, surgery, and antibiotics (within 8 weeks) with foul "horse barn odor"?
  - Requires ruling out *Clostridium difficile* ("C Diff")
- Age considerations?
  - Elderly patients may not present with classic signs and symptoms
  - Infants are at increased risk for dehydration
    - Number of diaper changes (e.g., wet or diarrhea) in past 24 hours
    - Best practice is to weigh a child without clothing up to age 3 years

- Questions to help determine amount of vomitus in a young child
  - Could you wipe the vomitus off the child with a diaper or rag?
  - Did it require a change of clothes for the infant or caregiver?
  - If it was on a bed, sheet, or floor how big a circle did it make?
  - Did it happen after every feeding?
  - Did it look like what was just eaten, or was it curdled?
  - What color was it?
  - Was the vomit projected away from the child?
- History of diabetic ketoacidosis (DKA)?
  - Up to 30% of new cases of type 1 diabetes mellitus are diagnosed when patients present with DKA identified from ketone bodies; ask about a history of "flu" in previous weeks
- Recent exposure to black widow (*Latrodectus*) spider bite?
  - Bite can cause severe muscle spasms in abdomen
  - Ask if the patient has been near dark, cool places that may pose a risk of a black widow spider exposure (e.g., a shed)

═══════════════════════════*FAST FACTS in a NUTSHELL*

- Remember that the bismuth from Pepto-Bismol and ferrous sulfate (iron) turn stools black. Stool with "digested" blood is stickier and has a foul odor.
- Atypical presentations can be "typical" in the elderly patient. Do not make assumptions regarding the origin of pain. Consider an atypical cardiac presentation in the elderly patient presenting with upper abdominal pain or nausea and vomiting. Look for the subtle clues. Approximately one third of patients older than 65 who are admitted with abdominal pain need surgery.

Generic Assessment

Vital Signs

- Abdominal pain with abnormal vital signs is usually more serious
- Signs of dehydration
  - Heart rate is more sensitive than blood pressure (healthy adult must lose 1,500 mL of fluid before exhibiting hypotension)
  - A pulse of 120 beats per minute or higher is highly indicative of dehydration or other serious illness

Skin Assessment

- Assess skin turgor on sternum or forehead where alteration in skin elasticity is less marked with aging

Abdominal Assessment

- Palpate the abdomen (consider peritoneal signs)
- Assess bowel sounds; initially bowel sounds can be hyperactive before hypoactive or no bowel sounds with an obstruction

Generic Interventions

- Anticipate the need for analgesics since early pain relief in stable patients with nontraumatic acute abdominal pain is recommended
- Anticipate the need to collect urine in premenopausal women for pregnancy testing even if they state they are not pregnant
- Consider whether an ECG within 10 minutes is indicated; refer to your facility protocol
- If suspicious of DKA, check blood glucose and send urine for ketones per protocol or physician order

FAST FACTS in a NUTSHELL

- Severe pain that is 7 or 8 on a 0-to-10 scale and lasts 6 or more hours is potentially a serious condition.
- Writhing or restlessness is also concerning as it is usually indicative of a colicky pain from stones.
- In the elderly patient, pain out of proportion to the exam should raise concern for the potentially life-threatening diagnosis of mesenteric ischemia.
- "Frequent" vomiting is considered to be 10 or more episodes in the previous 24 hours.
- An early sign of dehydration is a decreased ability to focus.
- Areas of the body to assess for dehydration include mucous membranes, tongue, or teeth (dry). Skin can be assessed for poor turgor.

SPECIFIC CONDITIONS

The questions, assessment, and interventions that follow are *not* intended to be comprehensive in nature but will help guide the triage nurse through the nursing process.

Cholecystitis

1. *Questions:* Time of last meal; history of recent fat intake; history of cholelithiasis; shoulder tip and acute colicky pain; presence of the 6 "Fs" (fat, female, forty, fertile, fair, flatulent)?
2. *Assessment:* Refer to Generic Assessment, earlier
3. *Interventions:* Give nothing by mouth (NPO) and anticipate the need for antiemetics

Pancreatitis

1. *Questions:* History of alcoholism or cholelithiasis; sudden knifelike pain in left upper quadrant, midgastric, or back (related to retroperitoneal location); is the pain worse with eating or lying flat?
2. *Assessment:* Check pulse oximetry (latent hypoxia is a major complication); signs of dehydration; hypovolemia (major complication)
3. *Interventions:* Anticipate the need for antiemetics and pain control

Peptic Ulcer Disease

1. *Questions:* Smoking history; taking nonsteroidal anti-inflammatory drugs (NSAIDs) or acetylsalicylic acid (ASA); gnawing or burning sensation intermittently?
2. *Assessment:* Vomitus for presence of blood
3. *Interventions:* Refer to Generic Interventions, earlier

FAST FACTS in a NUTSHELL

Patients with duodenal ulcers have reduced pain after eating while those with gastric ulcers tend to have more pain following a meal.

Intestinal Obstruction (Small Intestine)

1. *Questions:* Vomiting (gastric contents, then bilious, then brown fecal material); symptoms worse after eating; history of abdominal surgery (present in 50%–70% of patients)?
2. *Assessment:* Refer to Generic Assessment, earlier
3. *Interventions:* Refer to Generic Interventions, earlier

Intestinal Obstruction (Large Intestine)

1. *Questions:* Obstipation (feels the need to pass gas but unable)?
2. *Assessment:* High-pitched "tinkling" bowel sounds
3. *Interventions:* Refer to Generic Interventions, earlier

Incarcerated Hernia

1. *Questions:* History of intermittent "abdominal mass"; sudden pain with rapid increase in intensity; pain with bending over, lifting, and/or coughing?
2. *Assessment:* Palpate abdomen for "mass" that is now tender and tense
3. *Interventions:* Anticipate the need for surgical intervention

Abdominal Aneurysm

1. *Questions:* Abdominal or back pain, or both; sudden, severe tearing pain with radiation to groin; syncopal episode; male, history of smoking, or high blood pressure (increased risk)?
2. *Assessment:* Palpate abdomen for pulsating abdominal mass or rigidity; clammy skin
3. *Interventions:* Anticipate the need for rapid surgical intervention

Appendicitis

1. *Questions:* Pain starts around umbilicus and slowly moves to right lower quadrant (McBurney's point) over 48 hours?
2. *Assessment:* Anorexia; gait with limp; rebound tenderness with abdominal assessment; age considerations (most commonly occurs in those aged 11 through 35 years)
3. *Interventions:* Anticipate the need for surgical intervention

FAST FACTS in a NUTSHELL

Patients with acute appendicitis may experience delays in diagnosis or a missed diagnosis often due to vague initial symptoms including periumbilical and epigastric pain preceding right lower quadrant pain. Appendicitis does not only occur on the right side. The triage nurse should be aware that left-sided appendicitis may occur in patients that have an elongated appendix, situs inversus, or congenital midgut malrotation (Yang, Liu, Lin, & Lin, 2012).

Diverticulitis

1. *Questions:* Constant persistent pain (sometimes for several days); nausea, vomiting, and/or constipation; fever?
2. *Assessment:* Abdominal assessment reveals left-sided pain similar to an "appendicitis"; age considerations (symptoms typically after age 50 years)
3. *Interventions:* Refer to Generic Interventions, earlier

Testicular Torsion

1. *Questions:* Sudden pain (often described as "twisting" after sports activities)?
2. *Assessment:* "Saddle" (bow-leg) walk; unilateral, affected testis is usually firm, and tender; intense pain or minimal pain relief when the testicle is elevated; age considerations (most common in adolescent years)
3. *Interventions:* Anticipate the need for surgical intervention

RED FLAG FINDINGS

- Shoulder tip pain accompanied by abdominal pain (indicates free air from perforation rising and irritating the phrenic nerve)
- Acute colicky pain
- Pulsating abdominal mass
- Positive rebound tenderness
- Boardlike or rigid abdomen (from muscle contraction)
- Sudden-onset, severe abdominal pain
- Coffee ground or bloody emesis
- Bloody or black stools
- Severe pain that awakens a person from sleep

REFERENCE

Yang, C. Y., Liu, H. Y., Lin, H. L., & Lin, J. N. (2012). Left-sided acute appendicitis: A pitfall in the emergency department. *Journal of Emergency Medicine*, 43(6), 980–982.

20

Obstetric and Gynecological Emergencies

Polly Gerber Zimmermann and Lynn Sayre Visser

Patients seek care at triage for a variety of obstetric and gyne-cological presentations. Considering the worst-case scenarios and identifying not only those who are obviously seriously ill but those who might be is of utmost importance. The triage in-terventions for these potentially emergent presentations may be limited. However, knowledge and recognition of "red flag" find-ings helps the nurse advocate for the patient and potentially save the life of the woman and her unborn baby. This chapter provides a foundation for potential high acuity obstetric and gynecologic presentations that the triage nurse may encounter. See Chapter 19 for other presentations not addressed in this chapter.

Upon conclusion of this chapter, you will be able to:

1. State three obstetric and gynecological presentation worst-case scenarios
2. List three triage questions related to an obstetric and gynecological emergency
3. List three "red flag" findings of obstetric and gynecological emergencies

WORST-CASE SCENARIOS

Ovarian torsion, ectopic pregnancy, leaking amniotic fluid, ruptured membrane, preeclampsia, eclampsia/HELLP (hemolysis, elevated liver enzyme levels, and low platelet levels) syndrome, placenta previa, ab-ruptio placentae, trauma, prolapsed cord, emergency delivery, toxic shock syndrome, sexual assault

ESSENTIAL TRIAGE QUESTIONS, ASSESSMENT, AND INTERVENTIONS

Chapter 15 is a crucial foundation for the content that follows.

Generic Questions

- Fever?
- Nausea, vomiting, or diarrhea?
- Back pain?
- Vaginal bleeding?
- Vaginal discharge (foul smelling, color)?
- Urinary tract infection signs or symptoms (e.g., increased urinary frequency, sense of urgency, dysuria)?
- First day of your last *normal* menstrual cycle?
- Any chance you may be pregnant? (the answer "no" does not mean the patient is not pregnant; consider that the patient *could be* pregnant yet unaware)
- If pregnant, how many times have you been pregnant (gravida)? How many deliveries have you had (para)? Abortions? Number of babies expecting? Estimated date of delivery? Has your water broken? Any recent medication or drug use? Receiving prenatal care?
- Uterine irritability? Rhythmic contractions? If so, how frequent are the contractions and how long do they last?

Generic Assessment

- Palpate the abdomen
- Vital signs of the mother and, if pregnant, assess fetal health by fetal heart tones after the 12th week (110–160 beats per minute is an expected normal range)
- Fetal movement after 18 weeks (ask when the mother last felt movement; any change in fetal movement from normal)

Generic Interventions

- Consider analgesics per protocol since early pain relief in stable patients with nontraumatic acute abdominal pain is recommended (careful consideration needs to be taken with known pregnancy)
- Collect urine specimen for urinalysis per protocol or advocate accordingly
- Collect urine for pregnancy test per protocol in female patients of childbearing age, even if the patient believes she is not pregnant

FAST FACTS in a NUTSHELL

One patient's last menstrual period was 2 months ago but she adamantly said she could not be pregnant. *Denial is a powerful thing.* When asked why she believed she was not pregnant, she responded "Because I don't want to be!" (She was.)

The questions, assessment, and interventions that follow are *not* intended to be comprehensive in nature but will help guide the triage nurse through the nursing process.

Ovarian Torsion

1. *Questions:* Nausea and vomiting; low grade fever; severe, sudden-onset, unilateral lower abdominal or pelvic pain; pain that progressively worsens and radiates to groin or flank; abdominal bloating or swelling; pain with intercourse or exercise; undergoing fertility treatments; known pregnancy; previous ovarian torsion; known ovarian cyst or mass; previous pelvic surgery; history of pelvic inflammatory disease?
2. *Assessment:* Unilateral abdominal pain; unilateral rebound tenderness
3. *Intervention:* Anticipate the need for a transvaginal ultrasound and surgical intervention

Ectopic Pregnancy

1. *Questions:* Syncopal episode; missed or irregular period; minimal or absent vaginal bleeding; shoulder pain (Kehr's sign) with ruptured ectopic pregnancy; history of pelvic inflammatory disease (noted in 50% of women with ectopic pregnancies); sharp unilateral, lower abdominal pain that is moderate to severe and occurs around the sixth week of gestation?
2. *Assessment:* Evidence of shock following a ruptured fallopian tube
3. *Interventions:* Anticipate the need for a human chorionic gonadotropin (HCG) blood test and expect a positive pregnancy result; foresee the need for surgical intervention

FAST FACTS in a NUTSHELL

- A woman presenting with signs and symptoms of ovarian torsion requires rapid intervention. If the diagnosis is delayed, the ovary may become necrotic and the damage is irreversible. *Time is ovary!*
- An ectopic pregnancy is differentiated from appendicitis as the pregnancy test is positive. Anticipate the need for an HCG blood test as sometimes the pregnancy is too early to produce a positive urine test.

Leaking Amniotic Fluid/Ruptured Membrane

1. *Questions:* Presence of any urinary tract symptoms (e.g., dysuria, hematuria, increased urinary frequency); did you feel a trickle of fluid while standing or a gush of fluid when lying down?
2. *Assessment:* Determine if fluid is urine or amniotic fluid; amniotic fluid is odorless and colorless
3. *Interventions:* Anticipate the need to perform the fern test and Nitrazine (pH), or see if fluid gushes after lying down; if the pH is greater than 6.5, the membranes have likely ruptured

Preeclampsia/HELLP Syndrome

1. *Questions:* Vaginal bleeding; sudden weight gain (especially if in the face); estimated due date (more than 20 weeks pregnant is high risk); right upper quadrant pain; headache, visual disturbances, or altered mental status (presence may indicate edema in brain); multiple gestation, previous hypertension, obesity, or diabetes (comorbidities)?
2. *Assessment:* Blood pressure > 140/90 mmHg (highly significant); hyperreflexia
3. *Interventions:* Anticipate the need to perform a urinalysis per protocol and expect protein in the urine; initiate seizure precautions; transfer to treatment bed and position patient on the left side

Eclampsia

1. *Questions:* How long did the seizure-like activity last; what did the seizure-like activity look like; any associated injuries; estimated due date (more than 20 weeks pregnant is high risk); recent delivery; headache; visual changes?
2. *Assessment:* Examine areas of injury; presence of tongue laceration or broken teeth; hyperreflexia; fetal heart tones (do not delay initiation of treatment to obtain)
3. *Interventions:* Immediate placement in a treatment room; provide emotional support; initiate seizure precautions and protect from self-harm; anticipate the need for emergency delivery and magnesium sulfate infusion

Placenta Previa

1. *Questions:* Estimated due date (this condition is seen in the last trimester); vaginal bleeding (expect bright red painless vaginal bleeding); number of pads saturating per hour?
2. *Assessment:* Palpate abdomen (expect soft abdomen and no evidence of contractions); auscultate fetal heart tones (expect normal)

3. *Interventions:* Place the patient on her left side and limit exertion; anticipate the need for a pelvic ultrasound

Abruptio Placentae

1. *Questions:* Sudden, severe abdominal pain or cramping/contractions; vaginal bleeding (expect dark red blood); history of trauma, hypertension, or drug use (methamphetamine or cocaine)?
2. *Assessment:* Palpate abdomen (expect hard abdomen); auscultate fetal heart tones (expect abnormal fetal response)
3. *Interventions:* Transfer to treatment bed and position patient on left side; consider the need for oxygen and anticipate preparation for possible cesarean section

Trauma in a Pregnancy Greater than 24 Weeks

1. *Questions:* Mechanism of injury (refer to Chapter 26); vaginal bleeding or clear leaking fluid; contractions; movement of fetus?
2. *Assessment:* Consider rupture of membranes and presence of leaking fluid; monitor for uterine irritability and auscultate fetal heart tones
3. *Interventions:* Transfer to treatment bed and position on left side; if on a backboard tilt to the left; monitor for uterine irritability and fetal distress; anticipate the need to prepare for emergency cesarean section

Prolapsed Cord

1. *Questions:* Does the patient feel the umbilical cord protruding into the vagina (often experienced after amniotic sac breaks)?
2. *Assessment:* Visualize for umbilical cord presentation
3. *Interventions:* Position immediately in knee-chest or Trendelenburg position; place sterile gloved hand in the perineal area and lift the presenting part off the cord (do not move hand until advised by physician) and anticipate emergent need for intervention

=== *FAST FACTS in a NUTSHELL*

Every effort should always be made to maintain the patient's dignity and privacy. An emergent presentation such as a prolapsed cord requires immediate intervention to potentially save the life of the baby. Lack of bed availability is not an excuse for failing to validate that in fact the cord is presenting. Acting in the best interest of the mother and baby should always come first!

Emergency Delivery

1. *Questions:* Feels need to bear down or push with or between contractions?
2. *Assessment:* Bulging membranes visible at vulva or crowning of the fetal head; mother states the "baby is coming" or that she is going to defecate
3. *Interventions:* Apply gentle pressure on the crown to prevent rapid expulsion (support perineum to reduce tearing); allow head to rotate naturally; feel for the umbilical cord around the neonate's neck and unwrap if necessary once head is delivered; deliver the shoulders by guiding head downward (to deliver the anterior shoulder) and then upward (to feel the posterior shoulder); keep baby at level of uterus; vigorously stimulate infant, dry and warm; suction mouth and nose

FAST FACTS in a NUTSHELL

- In your triage career, you may find yourself delivering a baby in a car or waiting room. Availability of an emergency delivery tray at triage and access to bag valve masks of all sizes is imperative. Know where your supplies are and ensure they are always stocked.
- A third-trimester pregnant woman with hypotension and tachycardia or in spinal precautions needs to be positioned on her left side to aid blood return to the superior vena cava.

Toxic Shock Syndrome

1. *Questions:* Headache or confusion; high fever that began rapidly; recent use of tampons; vomiting or diarrhea?
2. *Assessment:* Rash (macular) with sunburn appearance that blanches with pressure; expect hypotension, tachycardia, and signs and symptoms similar to septic shock
3. *Interventions:* Initiate contact isolation precautions; position in modified Trendelenburg; anticipate the need for rapid treatment (e.g., intravenous fluid, laboratory and blood cultures, antibiotics)

Sexual Assault

1. *Questions:* What happened; when did it happen; where do you hurt; do you know who did this to you; were there any witnesses; were weapons involved; did you or do you want to file a police report?

2. *Assessment:* Areas of injury that can be visualized at triage should be assessed and documented; perineal assessment should be deferred until a person trained in sexual assault evaluations is available; determine medical stability
3. *Interventions:* Provide emotional support and reassure the patient that she is in a safe place; line of questioning should be in private and with nonjudgmental tones and gestures; notify law enforcement per jurisdiction protocols; contact the local sexual assault nurse or examiner per policy; clothing may be evidence thus any items removed should be placed in an evidence container per protocol (e.g., paper bag), labeled as evidence with patient name, and chain of custody instituted

================================*FAST FACTS in a NUTSHELL*

Ask about intimate partner violence during every interaction with a pregnant woman. Since the relationship between the woman and partner changes with the pregnancy, this period of time places the woman at a higher risk.

RED FLAG FINDINGS

- Imminent delivery
- Leaking amniotic fluid
- Protruding umbilical cord
- No fetal movement
- Abnormally high or low fetal heart tones
- Trauma in a pregnancy of greater than 24 weeks' gestation
- Pregnant with vaginal bleeding or passing large clots
- Seizures with known pregnancy
- Abdominal pain in early pregnancy
- Patient states "I was sexually assaulted" or "I was raped"
- Headache, visual disturbances, altered mental status, dizziness (edema in brain)

21

Psychiatric Emergencies

Anna Sivo Montejano

Triaging a patient with a psychiatric emergency is a common occurrence in emergency facilities today. Health care providers need additional knowledge and resources to handle this group of patients, because they may present with unique attire and mannerisms. For example, a patient may be wearing an antennae on his head, because he believes it wards off aliens. Being compassionate and respectful and not belittling patients is important. Professional demeanor goes a long way in setting the tone for an encounter with a patient experiencing a psychiatric event. This chapter provides a foundation for potential high acuity psychiatric presentations that the triage nurse may encounter.

Upon conclusion of this chapter, you will be able to:

1. State three psychiatric presentation worst-case scenarios
2. List three triage questions related to a psychiatric emergency
3. List three "red flag" findings of psychiatric emergencies

WORST CASE SCENARIOS

Suicide, overdose, psychotic episode, manic behavior

ESSENTIAL TRIAGE QUESTIONS, ASSESSMENT, AND INTERVENTIONS

Chapter 15 is a crucial foundation for the content that follows.

Generic Questions

- What can we do for you today?
- Has anything happened recently that was different? (e.g., trauma, medication noncompliance, etc.)
- New medications?

- Any history of:
  - A traumatic loss or exposure
  - Illness or injury
  - Secondary impact (e.g., loss of job, home, financial stressors)?
- Thoughts of harming self or others?
- Is there a plan to harm self or others?
- Sleeping habits (e.g., waking up often during the night, insomnia)

Generic Assessment

- Appearance (e.g., grooming)
- Affect, speech, behavior

SAD Assessment

The **SAD PERSONS** scale can be used to identify risk factors for suicide of adults and adolescence; the more categories the patient meets, the higher is the risk of the patient committing suicide.

Sex—gender; men are at higher risk due to more lethal methods
Age—older than 15 years of age
  - Adolescent patients have an increased understanding of deadly methods and access.
  - Adults older than age 65 are at greater risk; 70% of older adults who died by committing suicide had seen their primary care doctor within 30 days prior to their death (Eldelstein et al., 2009).
Depression
Previous suicide attempt or psychiatric care (prior attempts increase risk)
Excessive drug or alcohol use
  - Increased correlation between substance abuse and suicide
Rational thinking (irrational patients have an increased risk for self-harm)
Separated, widowed, or divorced
  - Social support lacking (specific for adolescence)
Organized attempt (specific plan)
No social support
  - Negligent parenting (specific for adolescence)
Sickness or chronic illness
  - School problems (specific for adolescence)

Each item in the SAD assessment correlates to one point for this scale. This assessment is one example; however, there are many variations.

- 1 to 2 points = low risk
- 3 to 6 points = moderate risk
- 7 to 10 points = high risk

Generic Interventions

- Ensure safety for patients and staff
- Remove any items that may injure the patient (e.g., belts, shoelaces, cords); place patient in a gown as soon as possible so belongings can be taken away and secured
- Provide emotional support
- Keep the patient safe by having someone watch him or her (e.g., security, sitter)

=== *FAST FACTS in a NUTSHELL*

- The Joint Commission National Patient Safety Goal 15 states that hospitals need to be proactive in identifying safety risks to their patient population. Any patient with a behavioral or emotional disorder requires an assessment to screen for suicide risk (The Joint Commission, 2014).
- Recognition is the first step in identifying high-risk patients so appropriate precautions can be taken.

SPECIFIC CONDITIONS

The questions, assessment, and interventions that follow are *not* intended to be comprehensive in nature but will help guide the triage nurse through the nursing process.

Suicide

1. *Questions:* Have you thought about harming yourself or others; do you have a plan to end your life; do you own a weapon; do you have anything with you right now that you can hurt yourself or others with; have you ever attempted to harm yourself; how are you sleeping?
2. *Assessment:* Self-care (e.g., hygiene)
3. *Interventions:* Refer to Generic Interventions, earlier

Overdose

1. *Questions:* What did you take; how much did you take; what time did the ingestion occur (if medication was ingested ask to see the bottle so you know the dosage and number of pills that may have been ingested); were you trying to kill yourself; why did you decide to overdose (for suspected or admitted intentional overdose); have you ever attempted to harm yourself before (if a "yes" response, inquire if the self-harm was an intentional overdose, etc.)?
2. *Assessment:* Refer to Generic Assessment, earlier

3. *Interventions:* Obtain all medications from patient and secure per policy; call poison control on every overdose or delegate if needed (intentional/accidental) per facility policy; think *absorption prevention* (i.e., minimize absorption of medication into the patient's body)

Psychotic Episode

1. *Questions:* Do you see or hear things that others around you don't; what do you hear?
2. *Assessment:* Refer to Generic Assessment, earlier
3. *Interventions:* Orient patient to the here and now; provide a calm, quiet environment; reassure; do not touch patient (patients may be out of touch with reality, hallucinating, and so on, and this may frighten them)

FAST FACTS in a NUTSHELL

Patients may exhibit symptoms of psychiatric illness when, in fact, the underlying issue is not psychiatric at all. The patient's final diagnosis may be thyroid storm, myxedema madness, serotonin syndrome, frontal brain tumor, neuroleptic malignant syndrome, steroid-induced psychosis, or an infection such as meningitis or encephalitis.

Manic Behavior

1. *Questions:* Tell me what you are experiencing; are you sleeping?
2. *Assessment:* Unable to sit still; talkative; restless; difficulty focusing; insomnia; flight of ideas
3. *Interventions:* Orient the patient to the here and now; decrease stimuli (e.g., limit noise)

FAST FACTS in a NUTSHELL

- Agitated, aggressive patients are unpredictable. When escorting the patient have the patient walk in front of you and tell him or her where to go. For example, "We are going down this hall to the room on the right." This allows you to keep your eyes on the patient and not become trapped in a corner or room where your safety is at risk.
- Patients who overdose may not be truthful. Don't worry if the "entire story" is hard to gather. Remain focused on airway, breathing, and circulation along with vital signs and assessment.

RED FLAG FINDINGS

- Patient expresses an intent or thoughts of dying or harming self or others
- Patient indicates he or she has a plan to harm self
- Patient arrives in possession of a weapon
- Patient admits to an intentional or accidental ingestion
- Aggressive or violent behavior
- Hallucinations (e.g., visual, auditory)
- Delusions
- Paranoia
- Speech is disorganized

REFERENCES

Edelstein, B., Heisel, M., McKee, D., Martin, R., Koven, L., Duberstein, P., & Britton, P. (2009). Development and psychometric evaluation of the reasons for living—older adults scale: A suicide risk assessment inventory. *Gerontologist, 49*(6), 736–745.

The Joint Commission. (2014). Hospital: 2014 national patient safety goals. Retrieved from http://www.jointcommission.org/standards_information/npsgs.aspx

22

Ocular Emergencies

Anna Sivo Montejano and Lynn Sayre Visser

People seek medical treatment for a variety of ocular conditions. Some presentations are straightforward while others may be more complex. What is important at triage is that the nurse rapidly identify conditions that pose a risk to loss of vision, and that he or she act with a sense of urgency. These presentations require rapid treatment and intervention in attempt to save the eye. Time is vision! This chapter provides a foundation for potential high acuity ocular presentations that the triage nurse may encounter.

Upon conclusion of this chapter, you will be able to:

1. State three ocular presentation worst-case scenarios
2. List three triage questions related to an ocular emergency
3. List three "red flag" findings of ocular emergencies

WORST-CASE SCENARIOS

Central retinal artery occlusion, detached retina, acute angle-closure glaucoma, chemical burn to the eye(s), penetrating trauma to the eye(s), blunt trauma to the eye(s), ruptured globe, foreign body/corneal abrasion, orbital cellulitis

ESSENTIAL TRIAGE QUESTIONS, ASSESSMENT, AND INTERVENTIONS

Chapter 15 is a crucial foundation for the content that follows.

Generic Questions

- Any visual disturbances (e.g., floaters, flashes of light)?
- Recent trauma (e.g., penetrating, blunt)?

- Eye protection with recent activity (e.g., welding, woodworking)?
- Use of corrective lenses (e.g., glasses, contact lenses)?

Generic Assessment

- Visual acuity exam
- Check pupils for equal size, roundness and reactivity to light, and accommodation
- Assess eye(s) (e.g., redness, drainage, corneal changes)

Generic Interventions

- If sudden loss of vision identified (e.g., partial, segmental, or total), notify provider immediately
- Consider the need for ocular analgesics (e.g., proparacaine), tetanus immunization, and give nothing by mouth (NPO) if anticipating surgery

FAST FACTS in a NUTSHELL

Patients with an ocular complaint should receive a visual acuity assessment, *but not if* they have sustained a chemical burn to the eye. For chemical burns rapid irrigation is the priority to halt damage to the eye.

SPECIFIC CONDITIONS

The questions, assessment, and interventions that follow are *not* intended to be comprehensive in nature but will help guide the triage nurse through the nursing process.

Central Retinal Artery Occlusion

1. *Questions:* Sudden, painless unilateral (e.g., partial, segmental, or total) vision loss; transient vision loss; feeling of a shade coming down over the eye?
2. *Assessment:* Pupil could be dilated with a decreased response to light in affected eye
3. *Interventions:* Notify medical provider immediately; anticipate need to rapidly reestablish retinal perfusion since irreversible

damage can occur within as little as 100 minutes of occlusion (Pokhrel & Loftus, 2007); breathe into a paper bag (causes vaso-dilation); anticipate orders for medications that lower intraocular pressure

Detached Retina

1. *Questions:* Visual field has a curtain or veil; seeing floaters or flashing lights; decreased peripheral vision; history of diabetes, sickle cell, nearsightedness, or previous retinal detachment?
2. *Assessment:* Refer to Generic Assessment, earlier
3. *Interventions:* Notify provider immediately since condition is time sensitive and potentially reversible

Acute Angle-Closure Glaucoma

1. *Questions:* Halos seen surrounding lights; cloudy vision; head-ache; nausea; sudden, severe unilateral eye pain; recently entered a dark room?
2. *Assessment:* Redness in eye; pupil slightly dilated and nonreactive; cornea opaque
3. *Interventions:* Notify provider immediately due to rapid need to decrease intraocular pressure

================================*FAST FACTS in a NUTSHELL*

Sudden atraumatic vision loss may not always be related to the eye. The triage nurse should routinely aim to see the bigger picture and not be misled by the patient who may be convinced "it's just an eye problem." Although the patient may have an eye complaint, the bigger problem may be an evolving stroke.

Chemical Burns to the Eye(s)

1. *Questions:* Name of agent? (alkali are worse than acids and cause liquefaction necrosis)
2. *Assessment: Do not* delay treatment to assess the patient's vision
3. *Interventions:* Anticipate the need for *immediate* irrigation of the eye. *Time is vision!*

Penetrating Eye Trauma

1. *Questions:* Object causing penetration (e.g., knife, pellets from a gun)?
2. *Assessment:* Refer to Generic Assessment, earlier
3. *Interventions:* Place an eye shield, stabilize object in place, and do not remove

Blunt Trauma to Eye(s)

1. *Questions:* Loss of consciousness; sudden loss of vision; trauma (consider head or neck injury)?
2. *Assessment:* Hyphema, check extraocular movements (mobility restriction due to muscle entrapment)
3. *Interventions:* Ice to injured area; place an eye shield to affected eye

Ruptured Globe

1. *Questions:* History of trauma (e.g., consider blunt or penetrating trauma)?
2. *Assessment:* Pupil is teardrop in shape and deviates toward the injury; hyphema; ocular pain and blurry vision
3. *Interventions:* Do not remove any impaled objects; secure object in place; if blunt trauma occurred, patch with an eye shield; patch the unaffected eye to limit consensual eye movement; anticipate surgery

Orbital Cellulitis

1. *Questions:* Recent sinus or dental infection; pain with eye movement?
2. *Assessment:* Pain with extraocular movements; impaired visual acuity (late finding); toxic appearance; fever
3. *Interventions:* Anticipate the need for a computed tomography scan of the sinuses and orbits, laboratory tests including blood cultures, and intravenous antibiotics

Foreign Body/Abrasion

1. *Questions:* Type of object; circumstances surrounding injury and time of injury?
2. *Assessment:* Pain may range from mild to severe
3. *Interventions:* Anticipate the need for analgesics per protocol (oral or ophthalmic)

- When testing visual acuity, check the affected eye first, followed by the unaffected eye, and finally both eyes. If the patient is unable to read the visual acuity chart, hold fingers up and record the distance at which the patient can see your fingers; ask the patient how many fingers you are holding up. Document this information.
- If the patient cannot see the letters or fingers, check for perception of shadows or light.
- The most common complication of orbital cellulitis is meningitis.

RED FLAG FINDINGS

- Cloudy vision
- Asymmetrical pupils
- Chemical to the eye(s)
- Visual gaze
- Presence of peripheral floaters or halos around light
- Presence of blood in the colored part of the eye
- Nonreactive or diminished pupillary response
- Seeing red or bleeding from the eye with one or more of the following: history of hypertension, bleeding disorder, trauma, or complaint of pain or change in vision
- Visual field as a curtain or veil
- Penetrating object to the eye
- Severe or persisting eye pain
- Sudden onset of changes in vision
- Total, partial, or segmental loss of vision
- Toxic appearance
- Steam burns to eye(s)
- Trauma to eye(s)

REFERENCE

Pokhrel, P. K., & Loftus, S. A. (2007). Ocular emergencies. *American Family Physician*, 76(6), 829–836.

23

Musculoskeletal Emergencies

Reneé Semonin Holleran

Patients seek medical care for musculoskeletal injuries resulting from numerous causes, requiring the triage nurse to determine if the presentation extends beyond the extremity or extremities. What may initially appear as a single extremity injury may in fact meet critical trauma criteria once more in-depth questioning occurs. This chapter provides a foundation for a few high acuity musculoskeletal presentations that the triage nurse may encounter.

Upon conclusion of this chapter, you will be able to:

1. State three musculoskeletal presentation worst-case scenarios
2. List three triage questions related to a musculoskeletal emergency
3. List three "red flag" findings of musculoskeletal emergencies

WORST-CASE SCENARIOS

Neurovascular compromise (e.g., fracture, dislocation), arterial occlusion, compartment syndrome, amputation, high-pressure injury

ESSENTIAL TRIAGE QUESTIONS, ASSESSMENT, AND INTERVENTIONS

Chapter 15 is a crucial foundation for the content that follows.

Generic Questions

- Location of pain?
- Onset (time) of symptoms/injury?
- What happened?
- Do you hurt anywhere else?

- History of diabetes? (Increased concern regarding sensation and poor healing)
- Tetanus immunization history

Generic Assessment

- Inspect the site of injury and remove dressings as appropriate; palpate for crepitus
- Observe for the presence of limb deformity or deformities and check circulation, movement, and sensation
- Assess the 5 "Ps" (pain, paresthesia, pallor, pulselessness, paralysis)
- Note pain out of proportion to injury or history
- Assess joints above and below the area of injury or pain
- Compare the injured extremity to the uninjured extremity

Generic Interventions

- Initiate cervical precautions if indicated
- Airway, breathing, circulation (control bleeding)
- Remove jewelry or restrictive clothing from the injured extremity
- Give nothing by mouth (NPO) if surgery/sedation is anticipated
- Anticipate the need for pain control

SPECIFIC CONDITIONS

The questions, assessment, and interventions that follow are *not* intended to be comprehensive in nature but will help guide the triage nurse through the nursing process.

Neurovascular Compromise

1. *Questions:* Mechanism of injury (e.g., fall, motor vehicle crash); when did this happen; any other injuries; numbness, tingling, or decreased movement of the injured extremity; ability to ambulate?
2. *Assessment:* Check circulation, movement, and sensation; palpate pulse distal to injury
3. *Interventions:* Splint in position of comfort; rest, ice, compression, and elevation (RICE); if loss of a peripheral pulse, facilitate rapid diagnostic evaluation including appropriate radiographs

Arterial Occlusion

1. *Questions:* History of a recent abdominal or joint replacement surgery; prolonged travel (e.g., airplane, truck driver) that required sitting for an extended period of time; if a female patient, history

of a recent pregnancy or delivery; pain with walking; history of prior venous thrombosis?
2. *Assessment:* Circulation, movement, and sensation; presence of redness, warmth, and extremity swelling
3. *Interventions:* Protect extremity from injury

Compartment Syndrome

1. *Questions:* Recent injury or surgical procedure to extremity?
2. Assessment: Assess the 5 "Ps" (pain, paresthesia, pallor, pulselessness, paralysis)
3. *Interventions:* Remove any external compression device after consulting with a physician (e.g., cast, splint); *do not* place ice or elevate the extremity (decreases circulation); initiate NPO status; anticipate an emergent fasciotomy

════════════════════════════*FAST FACTS in a NUTSHELL*

- If *pain is out of proportion* to the patient's injury or history, think compartment syndrome.
- When assessing circulation, always palpate a pulse distal to the injury.

Amputation

1. *Questions:* Time of injury; location of the amputated part?
2. *Assessment:* Appearance and extent of injury; signs and symptoms of hypovolemic shock (e.g., hypotension, tachycardia)
3. *Interventions:* Apply direct pressure and place a pressure dressing to stop bleeding; anticipate the need to position patient supine if signs of shock; if the patient has brought the amputated part (e.g., finger, toe, etc.), place it in moistened sterile gauze using sterile saline (do not saturate); place the amputated part in a plastic bag or container that is securely closed, label it with the patient's information, and then put the bag or container in ice water.

High-Pressure Injury

1. *Questions:* Location of the injury; what is the substance injected (e.g., paint, grease)?
2. *Assessment:* Refer to Generic Assessment, earlier
3. *Interventions:* Anticipate immediate surgical intervention (removal of the substance is vital to tissue preservation)

FAST FACTS in a NUTSHELL

- Loss of function of a limb or limbs can be indicative of a life-threatening problem.
- Good outcomes are often dependent on timely intervention.
- Wounds from high-pressure guns move down the sheaths of tendons and digits. Surgical intervention must be immediate so tissue can be preserved.

RED FLAG FINDINGS

- Pulseless limb
- Extremity cyanotic and cool to touch
- Loss of limb function and/or sensation
- Pain out of proportion to the injury
- High-pressure injury

Environmental Emergencies

Anna Sivo Montejano

The triage nurses role in environmental emergencies is to recognize "red flag" findings so the patient receives rapid medical treatment when indicated. The focus should be on the associated symptoms. This chapter provides a foundation for potential high acuity environmental presentations that the triage nurse may encounter.

Upon conclusion of this chapter, you will be able to:

1. State three environmental presentation worst-case scenarios
2. List three triage questions related to an environmental emergency
3. List three red flag findings of environmental emergencies

WORST-CASE SCENARIOS

Hypothermia, hyperthermia, cardiac arrest or injury resulting from electrical injury, submersion, life-threatening symptoms from bites (e.g., snake, insect, animal, or human) and stings

ESSENTIAL TRIAGE QUESTIONS, ASSESSMENT, AND INTERVENTIONS

Chapter 15 is a crucial foundation for the content that follows.

Generic Questions

• Number of areas impacted (e.g., bites, stings)?

Generic Assessment

• Assess site of injury (e.g., puncture wounds, drainage)
• Circulation, movement, and sensation as indicated

- Assess the presence of systemic complaints (e.g., abnormal vital signs)
- Tetanus immunization status

Generic Interventions

- Control bleeding if observed
- Remove jewelry or clothing from affected area
- Apply dressings as indicated
- Apply cold compress for animal, human, or spider bite
- Anticipate the need for pain control and antiemetics per protocols
- Use a marker or pen to outline borders of *localized* erythema and note date and time

FAST FACTS in a NUTSHELL

- When assessing a wound look for signs and symptoms of infection. Patients do not always arrive immediately after the injury occurred.
- If a human or animal bite, consider taking photographs per protocol.

SPECIFIC CONDITIONS

The questions, assessment, and interventions that follow are *not* intended to be comprehensive in nature but will help guide the triage nurse through the nursing process.

Hypothermia

1. *Questions:* What happened; temperature in the environment; exposure time; protective clothing worn?
2. *Assessment:* Core temperature less than 90 °F (32.2 °C); frostbite; burning, tingling, or numbness (fingers, toes, earlobes); waxy white color to skin or large blisters
3. *Interventions:* Initiate basic life support measures if indicated; core rewarming for a severely hypothermic patient: protect and do not rub parts that are injured; tetanus immunization per protocol

Hyperthermia

1. *Questions:* Temperature in environment; exposure time; any recent physical activity; has the patient been hydrating himself or herself?

2. *Assessment:* Core temperature higher than 105.8 °F (41 °C); nausea; vomiting; diarrhea; hot dry skin; seizures, altered level of consciousness
3. *Interventions:* Initiate basic life support measures if indicated; cooling measures immediately; rehydrate

Submersion

1. *Questions:* Type of water (e.g., salt, swimming pool, pond); duration of time submersed?
2. *Assessment:* Airway, breathing, circulation, disability impairment; temperature (possible hypothermia); rales or wheezing
3. *Interventions:* Initiate basic life support measures if indicated

Electrical Injury

1. *Questions:* Amount of voltage (e.g., low or high); duration of contact; hearing, vision, or speech problems; concurrent trauma?
2. *Assessment:* Any visible burn marks, entrance or exit wounds; check circulation, movement, and sensation to affected extremities
3. *Interventions:* Initiate basic life support measures if indicated; 12-lead electrocardiogram (ECG); dressings to visible wounds

Snake Bite

1. *Questions:* Type of snake, if known?
2. *Assessment:* Monitor the patient even if no pain or swelling noted
3. *Interventions:* Minimize activity and immobilize the extremity below level of the heart (decrease blood flow to decrease uptake of venom; Emergency Nurses Association, 2013)

Bites (Animal, Insect, Human, Tick, etc.)

1. *Questions:* Immunization status of animal (e.g., rabies vaccination); domesticated or nondomesticated (animal); recent hiking or camping trip?
2. *Assessment:* Underlying tissue damage (e.g., nerve, blood vessel); joint involvement
3. *Interventions:* Rabies vaccination as indicated per protocol (animal bite); ensure appropriate personnel follow-up with local animal control

Stings

1. *Questions:* Type of sting (e.g., bee, scorpion, marine animal)?
2. *Assessment:* If a bee or wasp sting, assess for a visible stinger

3. *Interventions:* If able to visualize the stinger, remove using a dull object to scrape away (avoid pinching, which will release the venom)

FAST FACTS in a NUTSHELL

A cut to the knuckle sustained from punching someone in the mouth has a potential high risk of infection. Obtaining a clear history of how the injury occurred can decrease the chance of a serious infection.

RED FLAG FINDINGS

- Seizure
- Altered level of consciousness
- Neurological deficits
- Chest pain, shortness of breath, dysphagia
- Suspicion of frostbite
- Febrile illness with systemic complaints
- Submersion
- Core temperature: extremely low (< 95 °F [35 °C])
- Core temperature: extremely high (> 105.8 °F [41 °C])
- Severe pain
- Electrical burn
- Severe muscle pain or cramping
- Change in circulation, movement, sensation of extremities
- Neurotoxic symptoms (e.g., cognitive impairment, numb or weak extremity, visual disturbances)
- Extended exposure to elevated temperature combined with physical exertion or dehydration

REFERENCE

Emergency Nurses Association. (2013). *Sheehy's emergency nursing principles and practice* (6th ed.). St. Louis, MO: Mosby.

25

Contagious Presentations

Anna Sivo Montejano and Lynn Sayre Visser

Patients with contagious illnesses who seek care may manifest a variety of signs and symptoms, often including dermal findings, which can be challenging to evaluate. The triage nurse's role is not to diagnose the rash, but rather to ensure that the patient's airway, breathing, and circulation (ABC) are intact and that potentially contagious conditions are identified and appropriately isolated. This chapter focuses on many conditions that are a high priority for isolation in order to protect the patient, staff, and those waiting.

Upon conclusion of this chapter, you will be able to:

1. State three contagious conditions
2. List three triage questions related to a dermal presentation
3. List three "red flag" findings of dermal presentations

CONTAGIOUS PRESENTATIONS

Chickenpox, shingles, lice, scabies, impetigo, measles, rubella; smallpox (a bioterrorist hazard)

ESSENTIAL TRIAGE QUESTIONS, ASSESSMENT, AND INTERVENTIONS

Chapter 15 is a crucial foundation for the content that follows.

Generic Questions

- Location of rash, wound, or inflamed area? (Ask about genitalia; the patient may not tell you)
- Pattern of rash presentation (e.g., begins on head first versus hands or feet)?
- Fever or sore throat?

- New detergent, medication, food, or chemical exposure?
- Exposure to others with a similar rash or anyone living in the same household with the rash?
- Previous rash or hives (and the cause)?
- School outbreak of a rash (e.g., scabies, lice)?
- Recent exposure to a person with a communicable disease?
- Recent travel (e.g., another country or region)?
- Immunization status: diphtheria, tetanus, and pertussis (DTaP); varicella (chickenpox); measles, mumps, and rubella (MMR); influenza; pneumococcal vaccine (PCV)?

FAST FACTS in a NUTSHELL

- On September 30, 2014, the first case of Ebola virus disease was diagnosed in the United States in a man who had recently arrived from Liberia. In the following weeks, two health care workers who cared for the patient contracted the disease and many other individuals were regularly monitored for symptoms. This case was a reminder to all health care workers that we must *always* be vigilant in assessing a patient's *travel history* in addition to questioning about symptoms, including fever.
- According to the Centers for Disease Control and Prevention (CDC, 2014a), the presentation of Ebola may appear as flu symptoms and include fever, malaise, headache, vomiting, diarrhea, weakness, or pain in the muscles or abdomen. In response to the Ebola scare, the Emergency Nurses Association (2014) encouraged a cautious approach to isolation, suggesting that all patients presenting with a fever be isolated and *then* additional screening and assessment should follow. Travel history should include asking if the patient has been to an Ebola virus region (e.g., Liberia, Sierra Leone, or Senegal) within the past 21 days or been exposed to individuals with Ebola or potentially at risk for Ebola.
- Isolation should include standard contact and droplet precautions in a closed door private isolation room. Refer to www.cdc.gov for the most up-to-date guidelines.
- Ebola spreads by direct contact with blood or body fluids of a person infected with the virus. These fluids include sweat, vomit, urine, feces, saliva, semen, and breast milk.
- Many diseases can spread from continent to continent or region to region when careful containment measures are not taken. *Always* consider isolating a patient who presents with a fever of unknown origin, and follow CDC and facility protocols.

Generic Assessment

- Characteristics of rash
  - Extent of rash
  - Appearance (e.g., macular, papular, vesicular, hives, etc.)
  - Color (e.g., red, blanchable/nonblanchable)
  - Distribution pattern (e.g., symmetrical/asymmetrical)
  - Examine hands and feet (may provide information that helps to identify the rash)
- Check mucous membranes for dehydration (e.g., mouth, eyes)

Generic Interventions

- Wear gloves while assessing patient to avoid contact with his or her skin or clothing
- Apply dressings for draining wounds
- Consider initiation of appropriate isolation for patient, staff, and visitors (e.g., airborne, droplet, contact) and use appropriate personal protective equipment
- Isolate patient if suspicion of a contagious presentation
  - Airborne precautions (e.g., negative pressure room, room with a high-efficiency particulate air filter); mask patient until placed in negative pressure room
    - Chickenpox/shingles (both airborne and contact precautions)
    - Smallpox (both airborne and contact precautions)
  - Droplet precautions: mumps, rubella (German measles), measles (rubeola)
  - Contact precautions: ice, scabies, impetigo, smallpox, chickenpox/shingles

FAST FACTS in a NUTSHELL

- Focus on the symptoms and nursing interventions *first*. If the dermatological findings seem allergy related, identifying the allergen is secondary to treating the patient.
- Rapid progression of a rash places a patient at higher risk for a severe respiratory condition and possible anaphylaxis.
- Early recognition of Stevens–Johnson syndrome and toxic epidermal necrolysis can result in quick, appropriate care. The patient may complain of a burning rash that begins on the face and upper torso, and skin can be noted to peel off in sheets. This patient presentation requires reverse isolation to prevent infection.

CONDITIONS REQUIRING ISOLATION

Many presentations require isolation to prevent exposure of other patients, visitors, and staff. The following discussion is *not* all encompassing but provides information that may help the triage nurse understand rash progression, determine when to initiate isolation, and guide triage decision making. For additional information see www.cdc.gov.

- *Chickenpox:* Occurs in individuals with a recent exposure to someone with chickenpox; patient may or may not present with a rash since patient is contagious 48 hours before rash erupts and remains contagious until lesions crust over; incubation period is 10 to 21 days after exposure to chickenpox (CDC, 2013a); rash appears first on the face, back, or abdomen and then spreads; rash starts as small red bumps (pimples) that develop into blisters and has varying stages of eruption; may have signs of dehydration from sores in mouth (due to difficulty swallowing fluids)
- *Shingles:* Occurs in individuals with a history of chickenpox; patient is contagious until the lesions crust over; rash does not cross the midline (follows a dermatome); extremely painful

FAST FACTS in a NUTSHELL

Shingles often only appear in one patch (along one dermatome), but if the rash is present along three or more dermatomes the nurse should be highly suspicious that the patient is compromised or immunocompromised (e.g., cancer, human immunodeficiency virus, recent transplant, taking immune suppressant medications). Shingles can include involvement of the central nervous system and may lead to potentially fatal encephalitis (CDC, 2014c).

- *Lice:* Rash mostly found on the scalp and behind ears, and patient feels movement on scalp (head lice); rash presents on waist, thighs, and groin (body lice)
- *Scabies:* Rash often found in the webs of fingers, wrists, belt or bra line, and buttocks; small black dot at the center of rash; severe itching; symptoms may not develop for 4 to 6 weeks after an exposure to scabies; patient can be contagious even before symptoms develop (CDC, 2010)
- *Impetigo:* Exposure to a person with impetigo; contagious until lesions crust over; rash to the lips, face, legs or arms and spreads easily; itchy blisters filled with yellowish fluid

- *Measles (Rubeola):* Recent exposure to a person with measles; incubation period is 10 to 12 days with rash appearing approximately 14 days after exposure; patient is contagious 4 days before rash erupts and continues for 4 days after the rash appears (CDC, 2013b); rash starts on the head before spreading to most of the body including hands and feet; three "C's" include cough, conjunctivitis, coryza (runny nose); Koplik (white) spots inside the mouth; causes itching; rash is said to "stain" the skin, changing from red to dark brown before disappearing (easier to see in light skinned people)
- *Rubella:* Recent exposure to a person with rubella; incubation period for 14 days after exposure; rash is first identified on the face and spreads to the chest, back, and limbs; lesions are in different stages of development; begins with fever, runny nose, and cough followed by characteristic rash; itchy
- *Smallpox:* Incubation period is 12 to 14 days; first week of the rash is the most contagious period; rash erupts first in the mouth, followed by a rash to the arms and legs, and later hands, feet, and other parts of the body; rash erupts all at once and appears uniform in size and shape; accompanied by fever, vomiting, malaise, head, and body aches

FAST FACTS in a NUTSHELL

- Does the patient have pain that lessens 24 to 36 hours after an injury and then rapidly worsens? Think necrotizing fasciitis, commonly known as flesh-eating disease. Symptoms tend to be rapidly progressive and may include fever, chills, nausea, and malaise. Approximately 25% of people with this condition will die (CDC, 2014b).
- Patients at risk for necrotizing fasciitis include those with a recent break in the skin (e.g., from surgical procedure, wound, or intravenous drug use), diabetes, immunosuppression, or a history of malignancy.
- The patient assessment may reveal *pain out of proportion* to what is visible on the skin and crepitus due to the release of toxins as tissue is being destroyed. Upon initial presentation, the wound may or may not appear infected but after 3 to 4 days the area of injury may appear purplish or necrotic (National Necrotizing Fasciitis Foundation, 2005).
- Although necrotizing fasciitis is not a contagious condition, a presentation of a reddened or purplish area with an accompanying fever should always cause the triage nurse to *consider* the need for isolation.

- Nursing interventions include anticipating the need for rapid medical or surgical intervention, antibiotics, and use of a marker or pen to outline borders of localized erythema and mark with date and time. Marking the skin helps staff closely monitor the progression of the area of concern.

RED FLAG FINDINGS

- Throat swelling, stridor, or drooling (new onset)
- Wheezing, shortness of breath, or chest pain
- Facial or tongue edema
- Rapid progression of symptoms or rash
- Mental status changes (confusion or decreased level of consciousness)
- New-onset petechiae or purpura with or without a fever
- Systemic complaints: near syncope, dizziness, shortness of breath, weakness, or nausea and vomiting
- Severe pain or itching
- Rash with severe headache, stiff neck, or fever
- Recent break in the skin with rapid onset progression (e.g., necrotizing fasciitis)
- Rash near the eye or vision changes
- Swelling and redness located near or around eye(s), over joints, or genital region
- Evidence of dehydration if immunocompromised
- Symptomatic with prior history of severe allergic reaction

REFERENCES

Centers for Disease Control and Prevention. (2010). Parasites—scabies: Frequently asked questions. Retrieved October 13, 2014, from www.cdc.gov

Centers for Disease Control and Prevention. (2013a). Chickenpox. Retrieved October 13, 2014, from www.cdc.gov

Centers for Disease Control and Prevention (2013b). Measles. Retrieved October 13, 2014, from www.cdc.gov

Centers for Disease Control and Prevention (2014a). Ebola (Ebola virus disease). Retrieved October 15, 2014 from www.cdc.gov

Centers for Disease Control and Prevention (2014b). Group A streptococcal disease. Retrieved October 9, 2014, from www.cdc.org

Centers for Disease Control and Prevention (2014c). Shingles (herpes zoster). Retrieved September 30, 2014, from www.cdc.gov

Emergency Nurses Association. (2014). A message from the ENA president: Ebola resources on the ENA website. Retrieved October 16, 2014, from www.ena.org

National Necrotizing Fasciitis Foundation. (2005). Get the facts. Retrieved from www.nnff.org

26

Trauma at Triage

Reneé Semonin Holleran

Trauma remains one of the leading causes of death worldwide. No person is immune from the potential of trauma and, unfortunately, trauma can even cause death before birth. Despite the fact that many countries have fairly well developed emergency medical service (EMS) systems, patients who have sustained a serious injury may present for care by private vehicle. When that happens, the triage nurse needs to be ready to identify whether the patient has a life-threatening injury or injuries. This chapter provides a foundation for potential high acuity trauma presentations that the triage nurse may encounter.

Upon conclusion of this chapter, you will be able to:

1. State three trauma presentation worst-case scenarios
2. List three triage questions related to a trauma emergency
3. List three "red flag" findings of trauma emergencies

WORST-CASE SCENARIOS

Airway, breathing, circulation, or disability impairment; penetrating, blunt, orthopedic injuries; burns; trauma (head, spinal, thoracic, abdominal, extremity, pediatric, geriatric); victims of violence

ESSENTIAL TRIAGE QUESTIONS, ASSESSMENT, AND INTERVENTIONS

Chapter 15 is a crucial foundation for the content that follows. In addition, an awareness of trauma criteria, which include physiological, anatomical, and mechanism of injury, is imperative for the triage nurse to determine the appropriate level of care for the patient. Not all criteria can be discussed in this chapter but "mechanism of injury" is elaborated upon because this is more commonly seen in triage.

The importance of posting trauma criteria in the triage area cannot be overemphasized. The ability to reference information quickly can make a difference in assigning the appropriate acuity level. Information about trauma criteria can be located at www.cdc.gov/fieldtriage/pdf/decisionscheme_poster_a.pdf.

Generic Questions

- Use trauma criteria (physiological, anatomical, and mechanism of injury) to facilitate line of questioning.

Mechanism of Injury

- Motor vehicle crash: Events surrounding the vehicle crash (restrained, ejected, high speed > 60 miles per hour, death in same vehicle, rollover, prolonged extrication > 30 minutes)?
- Involved in an explosion?
- Motor vehicle/cyclist impact > 30 miles per hour?
- Pedestrian impact?
- Fall: Adult > 15 feet; pediatric > 10 feet?
- Penetrating injury (e.g., gunshot, stabbing, etc.)?

Generic Assessment

- Obtain a *SAMPLE* history:
  Symptoms
  Allergies
  Medications
  Past medical history
  Last oral intake
  Events preceding the incident

Airway

- Patient cannot protect his or her airway; presence of blood or vomitus in the airway

Breathing

- Labored (e.g., accessory muscle use, retractions, nasal flaring)

Circulation

- Pulseless, decreased or absent peripheral pulses (check all extremities), pale and diaphoretic, pulse < 50 or > 100 (pediatrics > 120) beats per minute, uncontrolled bleeding

- Unconscious, altered mental status, loss of function of any extremity or extremities, bleeding from nose or ears, nausea and vomiting, suspected spinal cord injury

Generic Interventions

- Take action for any airway, breathing, circulation, disability, or environmental/exposure impairment
  - *Airway*: Open the airway with cervical spine protection and suction any blood or vomitus if present; initiate basic life support protocols if indicated
  - *Breathing*: Assist with ventilations as needed with bag-valve-mask; place patient on high-flow oxygen; allow patient to assume a position of comfort while protecting the cervical spine
  - *Circulation*: Initiate basic life support protocols if indicated; manage any uncontrolled bleeding
  - *Disability*: Assess level of consciousness
  - *Environmental/Exposure*: Remove any clothing and keep patient warm
- Decide which level of care the patient may require, for example, a trauma surgeon or care in the general emergency department.

═══════════════════════════*FAST FACTS in a NUTSHELL*

- If the triage nurse identifies a patient with a potential cervical injury who arrives by private vehicle, ambulates into triage, or is carried in the arms of a loved one, knowing where the supplies (e.g., cervical collar, backboard, etc.) are kept to enable immediate access is necessary. Calling for assistance from the local emergency medical services agency may be essential if extrication poses a challenge.
- Safety of the staff, patient, and others should always be the primary concern when managing a patient who has sustained an injury, especially one that is the result of violence.

CONDITION-SPECIFIC QUESTIONS RELATED TO TRAUMA

For the following worst-case scenarios, refer to the generic questions, assessment, and interventions at the beginning of this chapter for further information.

Penetrating Injuries

- *Assessment:* Head, neck, abdomen, pelvis, groin, and axilla

Blunt Injuries

- *Assessment:* Significant injury to a single region (e.g., head, neck, chest, abdomen, axilla, groin); patients with injury to two or more regions of the body

Orthopedic Injury or Injuries

- *Assessment:* Limb amputations and limb-threatening injuries, including loss of a peripheral pulse or a cold or cyanotic limb; serious crush injury; major compound fracture or open dislocation; fractured pelvis; fractures of two or more of the following: femur, tibia, and humerus; signs of shock related to these injuries

FAST FACTS in a NUTSHELL

Knowing which patients may be at a higher risk after sustaining a traumatic injury increases the nurse's awareness of a potentially worsening scenario:

- Age risk (younger than 5 or older than 55 years)
- Comorbidities: Diabetes, chronic obstructive pulmonary disease (COPD), cardiac disease
- Poor general impression of the patient: *"Looks like something is wrong"*
- Victims of violence: Sexual assault, domestic violence, child maltreatment
- Pregnancy of greater than 20 weeks' gestation
- Severe pain

Head Trauma

- *Questions:* History of loss of consciousness, how long; was there a period of "lucidity" and then a change in mental status; has patient taken anything that may have altered his or her mental status (alcohol or drugs)?

Spinal Trauma

- *Questions:* Able to move all of his or her extremities; any weakness; any complaints of neck pain, numbness, or weakness?

Thoracic Trauma

- *Questions:* Mechanism of injury (e.g., blunt or penetrating); respiratory distress; obvious signs of injury (e.g., open wounds, seat belt sign)?

Abdominal Trauma

- *Questions:* Mechanism of injury (e.g., blunt or penetrating); abdominal pain and, if so, where; any referred pain (e.g., shoulder pain, which could indicate a liver or splenic injury); nausea or vomiting; difficulty urinating or hematuria; obvious signs of injury (e.g., open wounds or seat belt sign); patient more than 20 weeks pregnant?

Extremity Trauma

- *Questions:* Open fracture or any open wounds near the injury; loss of function in the extremity; numbness or tingling in the extremity; loss of peripheral pulse?

Pediatric Trauma

- *Questions:* Was an appropriate restraint device used (if in a vehicle); abnormal behavior; parent concerned about any changes in the child?

Geriatric Trauma

- *Questions:* What medications is the patient taking; what other medical problems does the patient have (e.g., diabetes, COPD); what are the patient's normal neurological responses?

Victims of Violence

- *Questions:* Does the injury match the history or mechanism of injury; are you and the patient safe; is the patient intoxicated; is the patient accompanied by law enforcement; was the patient restrained during the violent act?

FAST FACTS in a NUTSHELL

- When taking care of victims of violence speak in a calm voice and ensure that it is safe for you and the team to approach the patient.
- Clothing and personal belongings may be used as evidence. Place items in an evidence container per protocol (e.g., paper bag).
- Use extreme caution when searching a patient who has been involved in a violent incident.
- Give weapons or evidence (labeled with the patient's name, date of collection) to the appropriate authorities or store in a safe area.

Burns

- *Question:* Has the patient inhaled any chemicals or been in an enclosed space fire?
- *Assessment:* Signs of inhalation injury including facial burns, singed nasal or facial hair; burns over a large area of the patient's body (> 20%); burns to the patient's hands or feet
- *Interventions:* Ensure that it is safe to approach the patient; patients with chemical burns may need to be taken directly to a decontamination area; use appropriate personal protective equipment; manage the patient's airway, breathing, circulation, and disability; remove all clothing and jewelry to stop the burning process

RED FLAG FINDINGS

- Obstructed airway
- Respiratory distress
- Positive loss of consciousness with a lucid period and is now unresponsive
- Patient with the following vital signs:
  - Glasgow Coma Scale < 14
  - Blood pressure < 90 mmHg
  - Respiratory rate < 10 or > 29
- Obvious penetrating injury to the head, neck, thorax, or abdomen

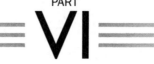

PART
VI

Special Considerations in Triage Nursing

27

Special Populations

Anna Sivo Montejano

Patients come to health care facilities seeking medical treatment. As triage nurses, our job is to assess them thoroughly, determine treatment needs, and direct them to the most appropriate treatment area. What happens when the patient has special considerations such as a hearing, visual, or cognitive impairment? Perhaps there is a language barrier, or the patient is a member of the military who requires special attention. How easy is it to thoroughly assess them and make sure that nothing is overlooked? Awareness of these considerations can make the difference in whether the patient receives the most appropriate care.

Upon conclusion of this chapter, you will be able to:

1. State three special populations seen by triage nurses
2. List two suggestions to improve communication with developmentally delayed patients
3. List three suggestions for recognizing a victim of sex trafficking

HEARING IMPAIRED PATIENT

When a patient with a hearing impairment arrive at a health care facility, we need to do our best to complete an accurate assessment. Simultaneously, we need to provide an environment in which patients feel their impairment is not affecting their ability to express their concerns and one in which our ability to understand them is not hindered.

Suggestions to Assist the Hearing Impaired

- Offer a certified sign language interpreter
- Use a paper and pen
- Have patients lip read if they state that is acceptable to them

- Pay close attention to nonverbal communication
- Use a text-telephone device (TTD) or telecommunication device for the deaf (TDD)

VISUALLY IMPAIRED PATIENT

A patient who is visually impaired requires the triage nurse to adapt the triage processes. Nurses may think they need to talk loudly so the patient can hear them. The patient is not deaf, so speaking in a normal tone when communicating is appreciated. Making patients feel comfortable when they cannot see their surroundings is an important part of reducing patients' anxiety in an unfamiliar environment.

Suggestions to Assist the Visually Impaired

- Introduce yourself and let the patient know everything you are doing; for example, "I am going to get a urine specimen cup for you"
- Ask patients if they need help before assuming they do
- Guide patients to where you need them to go by letting them hold onto your arm
- Let patients know how they can find you for any questions or concerns (e.g., if they are sitting in the waiting room, walk them to the front desk so they know where to find assistance)
- Update the patient verbally since the visual clues are not available
- Introduce every new individual involved in the patient's care; remember that he or she cannot see who enters the room
- If you leave the room, verbally tell the patient
- Ask patients where they would like their belongings so they know where to find them if an item is needed
- Make sure all their questions are answered and needs are met

PATIENT WITH A LANGUAGE BARRIER

Many languages are spoken in the United States today. With patients and visitors originating from all areas of the world, ensuring effective communication is vital. Treating each person as a unique individual and being respectful of differing beliefs can aid in recovery.

Suggestions to Assist the Patient With a Language Barrier

- Ensure that an interpreter is provided
  - Some facilities have in-house translation services

191

27. SPECIAL POPULATIONS

- Use a phone with two handsets so the patient and health care provider can be on the phone at the same time as the interpreter
- Utilize picture boards

Although convenient, avoid having family members act as interpreters. They may not accurately relay questions to the patient or convey all the information you provide.

DEVELOPMENTALLY DELAYED PATIENT

When a developmentally delayed patient arrives at your facility, how do you ascertain his or her level of knowledge? Where do you begin? How do you elicit the true story of the patient's visit? Health care providers are sometimes uncomfortable interviewing patients who are developmentally delayed. They may worry that important information may be missed, resulting in a detrimental outcome. In such situations, nurses must be careful not make assumptions. Family members, caretakers, and others who know the patient can help the nurse understand the patient's baseline function, assisting the nurse in performing an accurate triage assessment. The individuals who spend time with these patients know them best.

Suggestions to Assist the Developmentally Delayed

- Ask the accompanying person about the patient's baseline function
- Inquire about any changes the caretaker is concerned about
- Ask simple questions and move slowly
- Explain to the patient what you are doing
- Pay very close attention to nonverbal signs

================ *FAST FACTS in a NUTSHELL*

Patience is essential when meeting the needs of unique groups of people. Patients may not always understand what is going on in their immediate surroundings. Your patience and kindness can go a long way in facilitating the patient–provider encounter.

ILLITERATE PATIENT

An illiterate patient does not have the ability to read or write, which may not be evident initially at triage. However, paying close attention to nonverbal signs may provide clues. As triage nurses, we must clarify with patients, in a nondemeaning way, whether they can read and write.

Not following through when there is a suspicion of illiteracy can have detrimental implications because the patient cannot understand written instructions.

Suggestions to Assist the Illiterate Population

- Have the patient give you a return demonstration or verbalize key elements of discharge instructions
- Draw pictures to help with explanations or instructions
- Use pictures and pain scales (e.g., Wong–Baker) with assessments

MILITARY PERSONNEL

Being culturally competent in nursing has been a necessary ingredient to better understand the needs and values of patients of different ethnicities, socioeconomic status, religions, and so on, but we must not overlook another special population—our military personnel. The military culture focuses on loyalty, selflessness, and following moral codes. Nurses must be aware of the risk factors that military men and women are prone to so interventions can be timely and accurate.

Most Common Chief Complaints

- Mental illness (e.g., depression, posttraumatic stress disorder, suicide)
- Musculoskeletal conditions
- Postsurgical complications

The heightened awareness can assist nurses in asking appropriate questions and being aware of signs that might otherwise go unnoticed. The nurse may wonder, "Why doesn't the patient just tell me the real reason for the visit?" From a military perspective, a potential mental illness may serve as a major barrier to obtaining care.

Indications of Military Personnel (Former or Current)

- Tattoo of an anchor, eagle, or globe
  - Tattoo around the wrist (like a bracelet) that signifies a fallen friend from war
- Addressing others as "sir" or "ma'am"
- Clothing
- Body language

Do not hesitate to ask patients if they have been or are associated with the military. Such a simple question may make a difference in getting a patient the care he or she truly needs.

PATIENT WITH A LEFT VENTRICULAR ASSIST DEVICE

Health care providers are encountering left ventricular assist devices (LVADs) more often among patients with heart failure who are awaiting a heart transplant. Years ago these patients needed to remain hospitalized, but now these devices use battery packs that allow the patient to remain mobile. As triage nurses, we need to be familiar with the potential complications of these devices.

Complications in LVAD Patients

- Infection
- Thromboemboli
- Device malfunction
- Right-sided heart failure
- Hemolysis

Although knowing the potential complications is important, having a basic knowledge of the normal findings for an LVAD patient is also vital when completing an assessment.

Normal Findings in LVAD Patients

- Pulses are barely palpable or are weak
- Systolic blood pressure (SBP) range of 70 to 90 mmHg via Doppler reading
- Ventricular assist devices (VADs) "hum" loudly
- Be aware that these patients are on anticoagulation therapy

One must be familiar with the LVAD and understand the resources available to troubleshoot the device.

Suggestions to Assist LVAD Patients

- When assessing the patient, if there is concern about the device malfunctioning contact the LVAD center listed on the patient's VAD card (carried by the patient at all times)
- If you hear beeps or alarms, refer to the symbols displayed and call the number on the patient's VAD card
- If you need to assist with defibrillation or cardioversion, place the external patches, one anteriorly and one posteriorly
- Cardiopulmonary resuscitation (CPR) should be performed as a last resort, because the VAD can become separated from the aorta or apex of the heart during CPR

INTIMATE PARTNER VIOLENCE

Intimate partner violence (IPV), sometimes referred to as domestic violence, is an act in which the victim is assaulted by his or her intimate partner. The assaultive act may come in many forms. At times you may see a combination of these forms.

- Physical
- Emotional
- Financial
- Sexual
- Psychological

Recognition seems like it would be easy when one out of every three women have experienced physical violence from their intimate partners in their lifetime (National Intimate Partner and Sexual Violence Survey, 2010). Unfortunately, nothing could be further from the truth. IPV results in 33.5% of murders of women (Emergency Nurses Association, 2013) and affects not only women but also teenagers, men, partners in same-sex relationships (i.e., lesbians, gay), and bisexual and transgender couples. Recognition is the first step in helping victims of IPV.

Every patient needs to be screened appropriately since IPV is found in all of the following groups:

- Ethnicity
- Religious
- Economic
- Age
- Educational

The triage nurse must ask questions regarding the potential victim's safety, but the key is making these inquiries privately. If questions are asked in a safe environment and in a nonjudgmental fashion, the victim is more likely to be forthcoming about the history of the violence.

Sometimes the aggressor partner will not leave the victim's side, making it challenging to screen the victim. Explain to the patient that a urine specimen is needed, or an x-ray, thus separating the potential victim from the partner, in a location where the partner may not follow. This is your opportunity to ask the victim if he or she feels safe. Once IPV is identified, take action in accordance with your legal responsibility in the location where you work. Remember, you can make a difference in saving the life of a victim, but you must first ask the question.

SEX TRAFFICKING

Although sex trafficking is not an activity one would expect to encounter in the United States, sadly this problem is becoming more common. The term *sex trafficking* can refer to human trafficking (HT), commercial sexual exploitation (CSE), or child sex trafficking (CST). The vulnerability of children puts them at particular risk for this type of abuse. Victims are exposed to oppressive exploitation and physical and mental harm. Providing their "service" up to 12 hours a day results in physical injuries, sexually transmitted diseases (STDs), malnutrition, isolation, and psychological trauma. What can a triage nurse do to stop this horrific abuse? *Recognize* that this exists, *intervene* appropriately, and *refer* (Miller, 2013).

Suggestions for Recognizing the Victim

- Individual is accompanied by a person who stays close and speaks for him or her
- Individual lies about his or her age
- Inconsistencies regarding injuries and illnesses
- Individual does not have possession of his or her own documents (e.g., passport, birth certificate)
- Presence of STDs, yeast or bacterial infections, particularly in underage patients
- Highly anxious or obedient demeanor (Miller, 2013)
- Trafficker is often the same nationality as the victim
- Presence of tattoo that may be a number, symbol, or the trafficker's initials (shows ownership)

- Bald patches (e.g., hair being pulled out)
- Presence of a global positioning system (GPS) tracking bracelet (Peters, 2013)

One must be sensitive to what the victim is enduring on a day-to-day basis in a world with no hope of escape. Victims are often told by their traffickers that no one is there for them; they are alone. Consequently, they may have a distrust of others that incapacitates them.

Victims May Exhibit

- Fear and distrust related to possible imprisonment or deportation
- Shame
- Lack of emotion or, conversely, intense anger
- A strong attachment to the trafficker
- Anger toward the nurse or other health care professionals (e.g., the victim may fear that questions will upset the trafficker)
- Limited communication ability as they may not speak English
- Feelings of depression or possible suicidal ideation (Peters, 2013)

Tips for the Nurse

- Recognize behaviors that are characteristic of victims
- Talk to the victim *alone*
- Keep the victim and staff safe; interfering with the trafficker's "property" can result in an unsafe situation
- Notify security, local police, or both

A triage nurse's *awareness* is our first line of defense. With this knowledge and the passion to help the victims of this unimaginable slavery, we can make a difference in the lives of those who may not have come to the attention of victim advocates or child protective services in our communities. Do not think this issue exists only in faraway places. These individuals can be living in your community at this very moment.

FAST FACTS in a NUTSHELL

- Be mindful that a relative of the victim may be the trafficker. Trust your instincts!
- As triage nurses we must *look beneath the surface*. Every minute, every day, every patient could be a victim of sex trafficking (Peters, 2013).

REFERENCES

Emergency Nurses Association. (2013). *Sheehy's emergency nursing principles and practice* (6th ed.). St. Louis, MO: Mosby.

Miller, C. L. (2013). Child sex trafficking in the emergency department: Opportunities and challenges. *Journal of Emergency Nursing, 39*(5), 477–478.

National Intimate Partner and Sexual Violence Survey. (2010). Violence by an intimate partner. Retrieved October 22, 2014, from http://www.cdc.gov/violenceprevention/pdf/nisvs_executive_summary-a.pdf

Peters, K. (2013). The growing business of human trafficking and the power of emergency nurses to stop it. *Journal of Emergency Nursing, 39*(3), 280–287.

28

Pediatric Triage

Deb Jeffries

Wherever you may be working, it is imperative that you be prepared to care for the pediatric patient. Nearly 20% of patients seen in general emergency departments (EDs) in the United States in 2010 were younger than 15. Triage of pediatric patients can be intimidating for even the experienced nurse. Accurately triaging pediatric patients will require every bit of knowledge and expertise you possess with a little ingenuity thrown in. Always remember, when caring for children you really have two patients: the child and the caregiver.

Upon conclusion of this chapter, you will be able to:

1. State two high-risk pediatric presentations
2. Verbalize effective methods of communication with pediatric patients of varying developmental stages
3. Explain special considerations when triaging pediatric patients

PEDIATRIC TRIAGE: OVERVIEW

In spite of the challenges associated with triage of the pediatric patient, you are much more likely to make sound decisions if you fully embrace a critical concept: *Listen!*

- That's right: *Listen* to the parents or caregivers and fight with every ounce within you the temptation to categorize them as *overreacting.* Although you have no doubt heard it said that "parents know their child much better than you do," it bears repeating here: *"Parents know their child much better than you do."*
- *Listen* to the child. If children are verbal give weight to their words and learn developmental stages so that you will be able to communicate effectively with those of various ages. If they are nonverbal,

listen and pay careful attention to the intensity and pitch of their cry *and identify whether or not they are consolable.*

- *Listen* to your colleagues. Use the resources available to you whenever you are not comfortable with a presentation or are not sure what to do.
- *Listen* to the medical providers; ask questions. Often providers not only want to collaborate with nurses, they want to teach us, allowing us to become more expert.
- *Listen* to yourself. If your intuition "tells" you the child in front of you is sicker than the medical record seems to indicate, then do something about it and get that child in front of a provider.

DEVELOPMENTAL STAGES

Familiarity with developmental stages is a must. You cannot recognize abnormal findings if you do not know what normal is! While a full discussion of this topic is beyond the scope of this book, information applicable to triage assessments of children in different developmental stages follows.

Infant (Birth–1 Year)

- *Trust versus mistrust:* Separation fears begin at about 6 months; period of greatest growth; improving motor skills, from lifting head to standing

Toddler (1–3 Years)

- *Autonomy versus shame and doubt:* Likes the word "no"; separation fears continue; risk takers; negotiation with a toddler is not effective (*tip:* be friendly but firm!); allow child to remain with caregiver whenever possible; anterior fontanelles close at 18 to 24 months

Preschooler (3–5 Years)

- *Initiative versus shame and guilt:* Magical thinking is common; illness is sometimes seen as punishment; allow child the opportunity to ask questions; may want to dress/undress self

School Age (6–12 Years)

- *Industry versus inferiority:* Takes pride in accomplishments (*tip:* offer praise frequently); able to think logically (*tip:* explain what you are doing!)

- *Identity versus role confusion:* Independent, moody, risk takers (*tip:* allow them to have options whenever possible); excessively modest, despite of their appearance (*tip:* provide privacy when the patient is getting undressed; Newman & Newman, 2014).

══════════════════════════*FAST FACTS in a NUTSHELL*

- Communicating a caring attitude toward a child will make obtaining information from the parent or caregiver much easier. If a parent senses the nurse's frustration or lack of patience during the interaction, the subjective assessment will be much harder!
- It has been said that a teenager is a toddler in a grown-up body; they are both risk takers with similar fears.

INITIAL ASSESSMENT

The challenge of triaging pediatric patients stems from several key factors:

- Anatomical differences
- Developmental considerations
- Anxiety and fear in both the patient and parent or caregiver

══════════════════════════*FAST FACTS in a NUTSHELL*

- Children often present with signs and symptoms that are vague and nonspecific, and have the potential to suddenly decompensate.
- *All* children must be assessed upon arrival; failure to do a quick visual observation of young children, infants, and neonates can lead to devastating consequences. Consider the infant who arrives bundled in a carrier with a blanket over the top, and parents who state he or she "has a cold." Let's further suppose that, for whatever reason, there is a lapse of 20 minutes or longer prior to an assessment by a nurse. Imagine the horror of removing the blanket and finding a blue, apneic baby in the carrier.
- *All* children must be assessed upon arrival.

A rapid initial observational assessment tool is the Pediatric Assessment Triangle (PAT) (Chameides, Sampson, Schexnayder, & Hazinski, 2011). There are three components to the PAT:

1. General *appearance*: Level of consciousness, muscle tone, spontaneous movements, look/gaze, and cry
2. Work of *breathing*: Retractions (e.g., sternal, intercostal, supraclavicular), nasal flaring, positioning (e.g., tripod, head bobbing), audible airway sounds
3. *Circulation* to skin: Skin color (e.g., gray, mottled, cyanotic, pale)

The PAT provides the nurse with a general impression of the physiological status of the patient and assists the experienced nurse to appropriately prioritize patients. This assessment can be performed in any order and should not take longer than 60 seconds to perform. An abnormal assessment should prompt the nurse to facilitate immediate placement of the patient to an appropriate treatment area with the necessary resources at the stretcher side. (For additional information on the PAT, see http://tinyurl.com/q394pzh [Booth, Shirk, & Edwards, 2014])

The PAT is followed by:

- Primary assessment (airway, breathing, circulation, and disability)
- Secondary assessment (chief complaint and focused examination along with vital signs)

Although different throughput processes guide where and by whom this assessment takes place, the components do not change. This assessment process is completed by the head-to-toe assessment.

"See, I Am a Kid"

Part of the triage assessment process involves obtaining subjective data. Subjective data include anything the caregiver or patient tells you, often referred to as the history—both past history and history of current illness or injury. The mnemonic *C-I-AM-PEDS* ("*see, I am a kid*") was developed to ensure the collection of relevant data when assessing pediatric patients (Emergency Nurses Association, 2012a). Its use encourages a systematic approach to obtaining information, making it less likely that important details will be missed.

C   Chief complaint
I   Immunizations, isolation
A   Allergies
M Medications
P   Past medical history, parent's impression

D   Diet, diapers
S   Symptoms
(Emergency Nurses Association, 2012a)

A Word About Vital Signs

Any pediatric patient who will not be immediately placed in the treatment area should have vital signs assessed. Remember that "normal" vital signs do not always reflect physiological stability owing to the pediatric patient's ability to compensate. *Always* assess the patient to get a complete picture. Although numerous references provide vital sign parameters for various age groups, it is interesting to note the lack of consistency in the literature as to what defines the limits of "normal" ranges (Hohenhaus, Travers, & Mecham, 2008). Posting normal vital sign ranges at triage provides for easy reference.

There is a plethora of literature acknowledging the multifaceted vulnerability of pediatric patients; nowhere is this more evident than in the realm of medication errors. Therefore, all pediatric patients should be weighed in kilograms (using a kilogram-only scale). The weight should be recorded in an easily identifiable area of the medical record (American Academy of Pediatrics Committee on Pediatric Emergency Medicine, American College of Emergency Physicians Pediatric Committee, & Emergency Nurses Association Pediatric Committee, 2009; Emergency Nurses Association, 2012b).

═══════════════════════════*FAST FACTS in a NUTSHELL*

- A pulse oximetry reading is not necessary to determine acute respiratory distress. Assess work of breathing (e.g., seesaw respirations, use of accessory muscles, and nasal flaring). A child may be able to maintain a pulse oximetry measurement greater than 90% and still be in severe distress. Remember that *respiratory* compromise is the source of most pediatric arrests.
- Normal pediatric blood pressure is calculated using the following equation:

$$70 + (2 \times \text{age in years})$$

- A change in blood pressure in a child is a late finding.

Caution, Be on the Lookout!

Numerous symptoms should alert the astute triage nurse to a critically ill or injured child. (See http://tinyurl.com/lp8q949 for specific presentations applicable to the primary assessment of airway, breathing, circulation, disability, and exposure [ABCDE].) The Emergency Nursing Pediatric Course covers this content in greater detail. In addition to the presentations discussed in this chapter, anytime a child is reported by the parent or caregiver as behaving in a way that is unlike his or her normal behavior, pay careful attention.

FAST FACTS in a NUTSHELL

Use distraction techniques appropriate to the developmental stage of the child to accomplish your assessments. For example, an infant aged 6 to 12 months may be distracted by a brightly colored toy attached to your stethoscope while a 2 year-old may be more distracted by blowing bubbles with a wand.

PEDIATRIC PRESENTATIONS: TRIAGE PERILS

Apparent Life-Threatening Event

The presentation of an apparent life-threatening event is often assigned a lower acuity level at triage because the infant looks "just fine" upon arrival. Do not be fooled; any infant with a reported episode of apnea, color change, change in muscle tone, accompanied by choking or gagging is a high acuity patient. Anticipate the immediate need for continuous cardiac and pulse oximetry monitoring. Parents often describe an episode in which they believed that the infant had died.

Foreign Body Aspiration/Obstruction

Young children like to put anything and everything into their mouths. Foreign body aspiration is most common in children younger than age 3 years. If a young child presents with sudden onset of respiratory distress without a known precipitating event, think possible foreign body aspiration or obstruction.

Croup

Croup is a very common childhood illness in which upper airway obstruction occurs due to inflammation and swelling. By the time stridor is present, significant airway swelling has occurred. Anticipate the need for humidified blow-by oxygen, dexamethasone, and nebulized racemic epinephrine.

Bronchiolitis

A very common condition in young children and infants, bronchiolitis represents a constellation of infections, the most common of which is respiratory syncytial virus (RSV). RSV occurs most often in winter and early spring, especially in very young or premature infants and can be life threatening. Be prepared for frequent nasal suctioning, especially in obligate nose breathers. Moving them out of triage as soon as you are able is a good idea.

Fever

Fever accompanies a wide range of illnesses, from minor to life threatening. When assessing children remember that fever, or lack thereof, does not necessarily indicate severity of illness. A child can be hypothermic, normothermic, or hyperthermic and be critically ill.

Nursemaid's Elbow

With nursemaid's elbow, subluxation of the radial head occurs after forceful jerking of the arm (e.g., being pulled by the arm). The child holds the arm in a position of comfort and typically refuses to use it. Think mechanism of injury with this one!

Child Abuse

Knowledge of developmental stages is important in order to detect when a child is being abused or neglected. Be very attuned to injuries that are inconsistent with developmental stages or history. For example, it is extremely unlikely that a 6-month-old fell and sustained a femur fracture while walking. On the other hand, bruising to a 2-year-old's shins is common as they often fall as they toddle about. A full discussion of child abuse and neglect is beyond the scope of this chapter, but always remember you *must* report suspected child abuse to the authorities. Do not assume that another provider or social worker is reporting suspected abuse. As nurses, we are expected to report it as well. We are all mandated reporters.

- Drooling that is inappropriate for the age of the patient is a "red flag" that should get your immediate attention.
- Any neonate (0–28 days) with a fever of 100.4 °F (38 °C) or greater is a high acuity patient.
- If a baby is excessively crying without an apparent reason, check the fingers, toes, and penis for a hair tourniquet.

REFERENCES

American Academy of Pediatrics Committee on Pediatric Emergency Medicine, American College of Emergency Physicians Pediatric Committee, & Emergency Nurses Association Pediatric Committee. (2009). Joint policy statement—Guidelines for care of children in the emergency department. *Pediatrics, 124*(4), 1233–1243.

Booth, J. S., Shirk, A., Edwards, A. R. (2014). Pediatric Resuscitation. Retreived from http://tinyurl.com/q394pzh

Chameides, L., Sampson, R. A., Schexnayder, S. M., & Hazinski M. F. (Eds.). (2011). *Pediatric advanced life support provider manual*. Dallas, TX: American Heart Association.

Emergency Nurses Association. (2012a). *Emergency nursing pediatric course provider manual* (4th ed.). Des Plaines, IA: Author.

Emergency Nurses Association. (2012b). *Position statement: Weighing pediatric patients in kilograms*. Retrieved from http://www.ena.org/SiteCollectionDocuments/Position%20Statements/WeighingPedsPtsinKG.pdf

Hohenhaus, S., Travers, D., & Mecham, N. (2008). Pediatric triage: A review of emergency education literature. *Journal of Emergency Nursing, 34*(4), 308–313.

Newman, B., & Newman, P. (2014). *Development through life: A psychosocial approach* (12th ed.). Independence, KY: Cengage Learning.

29

Geriatric Triage

Anna Sivo Montejano

Today there are more people than ever before over the age of 65 years. By the year 2050, projections are that one out of five Americans will be older than 65 (Touhy & Jett, 2012). As a result of this expanding population of older Americans, many facilities see increased numbers of elderly patients who are seeking medical care for their complaints. Special consideration should be given to this population because they may arrive with atypical presentations that can be overlooked in the triage arena, putting the patient at risk for deterioration or even death. Gathering information relevant to the elderly patient's complaint can be challenging because of possible sensory deficits or physical limitations. A keen eye and patience will allow the nurse to gather the information needed to assign an accurate acuity level and facilitate the most appropriate disposition following triage.

Upon conclusion of this chapter, you will be able to:

1. State three physical changes that occur to the elderly
2. State three types of violence against the elderly population
3. Explain an atypical presentation

GERIATRIC ASSESSMENT

As people become older, physiological changes occur throughout the body, including respiratory, cardiovascular, and musculoskeletal systems. This is an ongoing process as we age. When performing a physical assessment, an awareness of these physiological changes is important since the changes put the patient at risk for additional problems (e.g., dehydration).

Some Physical Changes

- Sensory and motor impairment
  - Hearing and vision
  - Touch, pain, and temperature

- Skin
  - Decreased blood supply
  - Increased fragility
- Decreased subcutaneous tissue
- Decreased contractility and heart rate
- Decreased lung capacity
- Decreased kidney function

Some Emotional Changes

- Depression
  - Loss of significant other (e.g., living alone)
  - Loss of friends
- Caregiver role fatigue
  - When caring for an elderly spouse (e.g., an 80-year-old wife with a physically or mentally disabled 83-year-old husband may be "on call" as the primary caretaker 24/7)

Potential Risks

- Malnutrition
- Dehydration
- Cardiovascular disease
  - Remains the leading cause of death in adults older than age 85 (Lewis, Dirksen, & Heitkemper, 2011).
- Medication interaction

Critical thinking and application of geriatric knowledge can decrease the patient's risk for a poor outcome by leading to early initiation of needed interventions.

FAST FACTS in a NUTSHELL

- Elderly patients often delay seeking help for their problems, alerting the nurse to consider a higher acuity level when they do present with health complaints.
- If you need to remove an article of clothing while assessing the elderly patient (e.g., to take a blood pressure reading), complete the task as quickly as possible to minimize his or her discomfort (e.g., feeling cold).

COMMUNICATING WITH A GERIATRIC PATIENT

Assessing the geriatric population relies on the nurse's critical thinking and decision-making skills. Often elderly patients will not seek help until it is absolutely necessary or their loved ones force them to be evaluated. Many elderly are independent and self-sufficient and fear having that independence taken away. When communicating with these individuals, be aware of their feelings and express compassion about their concerns. The triage process typically takes more time when caring for the elderly; be patient. Rushing elderly patients often prolongs the process as they may become easily flustered.

Reasons for Communication Delays

- Possible short-term memory loss
  - Recalling the specifics for the visit may offer challenges
- Perception is that they will be seen quickly and then released
- Many questions asked by multiple people causes:
  - Frustration
  - Irritation
  - Misunderstanding (especially if English is not their first language)
- Their need to return home quickly to care for a loved one or animal is of high priority

Tips for Effective Communication With the Geriatric Population

- Speak slowly and clearly
- Do not ask too many questions at once
- If the patient is hard of hearing, speak in a lower tone of voice
- Provide reassurance
- Do not refer to the patient as "honey," "sweetie," or in similar terms
  - These words can be interpreted as disrespectful or condescending
- Keep your promises
- Be honest
- Recognize that there may be a delay in obtaining information in triage
  - Some patients may tell you more than you need to know, including details of a vacation or about a family member who had similar symptoms years ago
  - Patients may have brought numerous medications for the nurse to sort through

- Allow the patient to make choices, even if small ones
  - "Where do you want me to put your eyeglasses?
- Ask for permission if you need to assist in removing an article of clothing

Geriatric patients can be set in their ways and particular about how their personal possessions are handled or put away. Be respectful and conscious of their concerns. Certain personal items may be expensive or sentimental. A health care provider who attempts to remove or displace these items can cause anxiety.

Examples of Items of Concern to the Elderly

- Keys
- Medications
- Purse or wallet
- Eyeglasses
- Dentures
- Medical cards

EXAMINATION TIPS

The following simple examination tips can facilitate the assessment, making the process a relatively easy experience instead of an anxiety-provoking one (for the patient) and lengthy (for the nurse or physician).

Suggestions for the Geriatric Examination in Triage

- Only expose areas being examined; geriatric patients get cold easily
- Provide warm blankets if able
- Assist the patient with removal of clothing if needed; ask for permission to do so
- Ask closed ended questions
  - Questions that require only "yes" or "no" answers limit the discussion of unnecessary information

POLYPHARMACY

Polypharmacy, a situation in which a patient is using multiple medications, often occurs in the elderly population. It can cause adverse drug reactions that may go unnoticed by the treating physician or lead to additional medications being prescribed to treat the patient's new complaint. However, these additional medications can, in turn, cause further drug-related problems.

- Clonidine
- Cyclobenzaprine
- Diazepam
- Diphenhydramine
- Hydroxyzine
- Ketorolac
- Meperidine
- Nifedipine
- Promethazine
- Propoxyphene (Donatelli & Somes, 2013)

As triage nurses we must be alert for elderly patients who present to the triage area with complaints such as confusion or dizziness. The nurse's first thought may be that the patient is experiencing a neurological issue, but a complete medication history, including over-the-counter medications, and a heightened awareness of drug reactions may lead to a different conclusion.

ATYPICAL PRESENTATION

An atypical presentation, simply defined, is one that does not manifest with expected symptoms and signs. Atypical presentations can result in missed diagnoses, and this issue is of particular concern in elderly patients because their complaints are often vague or nonspecific. For example, an acute myocardial infarction is often misdiagnosed or overlooked because the elderly patient arrives with a complaint of general weakness, epigastric discomfort, or confusion. As health care providers, we are listening for classic descriptions like chest pain, nausea, or diaphoresis. The presence of risk factors (e.g., diabetes) should increase the nurse's awareness that the patient may be in danger. Recognizing and appropriately intervening can make a difference in the patient's outcome.

ELDER ABUSE

Elderly patients are at risk for abuse due to their vulnerability and dependence on others for help. Unfortunately, all too often a trusted individual is the abuser.

Types of Abuse

- Physical
- Neglect

- Psychological
- Sexual
- Financial
- Abandonment

Be aware of this worldwide phenomenon and take time to listen to your patients. If you receive any information that raises your suspicions that elder abuse may be occurring follow through and notify appropriate personnel. Your actions may contribute to stopping the abuse. Recognition of an abusive situation while a patient is in your care may be the patient's only chance for intervention.

FAST FACTS in a NUTSHELL

Elder abuse goes largely unreported. The key to identifying abuse is to use all of your senses and to recognize that this problem occurs in all settings and at all societal levels.

CULTURAL COMPETENCE

Today's nurses will most likely deliver care to patients who are of a different culture, reinforcing the need for culturally competent care. It is expected that by the year 2050, the groups currently designated as minorities in the United States will become the majority (Touhy & Jett, 2012). Cultural competence includes an awareness not only of our own personal values and beliefs but also those of other individuals in our community.

In certain cultures, pain is not expressed outwardly. If a patient presents to triage with a complaint of chest pain but appears calm and without pain, the nurse may interpret this symptom as "no big deal." This interpretation may erroneously lead us to believe that the patient is stable because he or she is not exhibiting signs of pain or distress. As a result, the patient may be assigned a lower than warranted acuity level leading to an inappropriate disposition.

FAST FACTS in a NUTSHELL

If a nurse is unaware of cultural differences and approaches patients as if everyone responds the same to any given situation, an inaccurate acuity designation may be assigned, resulting in a negative outcome.

Donatelli, N. S., & Somes, J. (2013). Beer list: What's NOT on "tap" for the older adult? *Journal of Emergency Nursing, 39*(5), 491–494.

Lewis, S. L., Dirksen, S. R., & Heitkemper, M. M. (2011). *Medical–surgical nursing: Assessment and management of clinical problems* (8th ed.). St. Louis, MO: Elsevier.

Touhy, T. A., & Jett, K. (2012). Ebersole & Hess' *toward healthy aging: Human needs and nursing response* (8th ed.). St. Louis, MO: Elsevier.

30

Patient and Staff Safety

Anna Sivo Montejano

Violence seems to be everywhere in our society. News media and newspapers are saturated with stories of violent acts, and you may have experienced violence personally or professionally yourself. As a triage nurse, you are highly vulnerable to both verbal and physical forms of violence. Since the triage area is often set apart from the rest of the department, isolation and seclusion are real concerns. The patient volume of the facility may dictate the number of resources present at triage. For example, a rural emergency department (ED) may have only one triage nurse who also functions as the charge nurse and a staff nurse, whereas higher census facilities may have multiple staff at triage. No matter the size of the facility, one common theme is that the occurrence of violence is inevitable.

Upon conclusion of this chapter, you will be able to:

1. Identify what causes a patient to become agitated, which can lead to violence
2. State two types of violence
3. Identify three ways to provide a safe environment

TYPES OF VIOLENCE

- *Verbal abuse* is one form, which consists of yelling, swearing, threatening, accusing, intimidating, making demands, or simply raising one's voice
- *Physical abuse* is the attacking of an individual or threatening the person physically; it includes physically throwing objects from small items like a pencil to large items like a wheelchair; at times there is biting, spitting, grabbing, punching—the list goes on

POTENTIAL FOR VIOLENCE

What makes a person violent? Often nurses wonder why anyone would be violent toward us. After all, we are here to help patients recover from their illness or injury. Why do some people begin yelling before we are given a chance to show them how nice we are? Why do they become angry when we are not able to take them to a bed immediately upon their arrival? Do patients not realize our resources are limited, and theirs is just one of the nearly 120 million ED visits that occur annually in the United States? Recognizing that some individuals have characteristics that increase their chances of becoming violent while others are influenced by situational or environmental factors is important.

Qualities of a Potentially Violent Patient or Visitor

- Intimidating
- Threatening
- Brisk pace
- Mumbling
- Loud speech; demanding
- Using profanity
- Rapid speech
- Entering another individual's personal space
- Throwing objects
- Under the influence of drugs or alcohol

Situational Reasons for Agitation

- *Miscommunication.* Imagine an elderly parent with complaints of fever and vomiting. The daughter calls the physician, who tells her to go directly to the ED, where "there will be a bed waiting for your mother." When the family arrives at the ED the triage nurse informs them that there is no bed available, and the ED has not received a call from the physician. Due to this initial miscommunication there is an increased chance that the daughter (or another accompanying family member) may exhibit frustration or agitation toward the triage nurse.
- *Crowded waiting room.* A patient presents for medical care and finds the waiting room (WR) packed. The line of people wanting to be seen flows from the front desk out the door and into the hall. People occupy all the waiting room chairs, wheelchairs obstruct the staff's ability to walk, and some of those waiting are even sprawled on the

floor. This sight alone can be overwhelming, even without the noises and smells experienced upon entering the WR. The patient quickly realizes that the chances of being seen in a short period of time are extremely slim. In this situation, the sights, sounds, smells, and the likely lengthy time it will take to be seen can combine to increase his or her anxiety, resulting in agitation and the potential for violence.

- *Ambulance arrival.* A patient is transported to the hospital by ambulance only to be sent to the WR. Envision the patient's arrival: the gurney is brought out to triage and the patient is unloaded. As a triage nurse, this does not faze you in the least. This practice is common in facilities that handle large numbers of patients. Those with low acuity complaints are often taken to triage. However, this can be extremely frustrating to the patient, who may have expected to be placed in a bed upon arrival. The patient may respond by using abusive language and may become agitated.

- *Insurance.* Some patients who have insurance assume they will be seen before those who are uninsured.

  - Example: A male patient with insurance arrives at the ED with a complaint of a laceration to the finger after opening a box with a box cutter. Five minutes later an uninsured, homeless man arrives with complaints of ischemic chest pain. The triage nurse takes the homeless patient with chest pain to the treatment area first. Visibly upset, the first patient approaches the triage nurse and, leaning forward into the nurses' personal space, loudly verbalizes that because he has insurance and arrived first he should be given priority.

- *Patients comparing themselves to others with the same complaint.* Occasionally two patients arrive with seemingly identical complaints, but the person who arrives later is taken for evaluation before the earlier-arriving patient.

  - Example: Patient "A" arrives with her significant other, complaining of a migraine. Your comprehensive assessment shows normal vital signs, no neurological deficits, no past medical history, and no reported allergies. The patient has self-diagnosed herself with a migraine. Patient "B" arrives also complaining of a migraine. After completing the comprehensive assessment, the nurse is concerned because of the patient's history of breast cancer and her report that this headache "feels different" than her usual migraines. Patient "B" is brought for evaluation first. Patient "A," or her significant other, may become angry because of their perception of the situation. The triage nurse should be aware that agitation may ensue.

Ways in Which ED Staff Play a Role in Increased Patient/Visitor Agitation

- Restricting the patient's choice
  - Example: Not allowing a patient to drink or eat, but failing to explain why
- Restricting visitation
- Not keeping one's promise
  - Example: Visitors would like to see their mother, who is a patient in the ED. They are told someone will come and get them in "a minute." Thirty minutes later they are still waiting.
- Denying a comfort measure
  - Example: A patient or visitor requests a warm blanket or a cup of coffee and is denied the requested item without an explanation.
- Making promises and not following through
- Communicating incongruently (e.g., verbal communication does not match nonverbal communication)
- Failing to provide information or reassessment, or both
  - Example: A patient has been waiting 3 hours to be seen by a provider. No update or information is provided about the wait time, nor is a reassessment completed by the triage nurse. This lack of information or compassion may result in increased agitation.

FAST FACTS in a NUTSHELL

- The key to decreasing violence in the triage area is *prevention*. Assessing the risks for agitation, including behavior, environment, and the staff's role, can help in de-escalating a situation before it progresses to violence.
- Staff education in management of aggressive behavior (MOAB) is a must. Additional information can be obtained at www.moabtraining.com/main.php. In addition, the Emergency Nurses Association provides a toolkit on workplace violence at http://www.ena.org/practiceresearch/Practice/ViolenceToolKit/Documents/toolkitpg7.htm

PSYCHIATRIC PATIENTS

Psychiatric conditions can be a factor in agitation leading to violence. Many patients arrive at triage with some level of psychosocial emergency. Those with a history of psychiatric illness may have trouble processing external stimuli and are often less able to handle the environment of the ED. Additionally, they may not understand why they do not receive immediate care. Some aspects of their illness make it difficult to think rationally, which may increase the tendency to react with violence. Triage nurses must be able to differentiate patients who are restless, irritable, or having hallucinations (e.g., auditory, visual), and those who may be a danger to themselves or others, and respond in a caring and sensitive manner.

ALCOHOL AND SUBSTANCE ABUSE

Alcohol, drugs, and illicit substances that are used separately or in combination can create a volatile situation when an impaired patient is brought to triage. The triage nurse must have a heightened aware-ness of the risks in this situation to stay safe and keep the patient safe. When interacting with an individual who is under the influence of alcohol or drugs, the triage nurse must pay close attention to the person's verbal responses. The patient may be loud, use foul language, and may encroach on the nurse's personal space, causing the nurse to feel uncomfortable.

Imagine a crowded waiting room in which a patient under the influence of alcohol starts yelling loudly about his disapproval of the wait time. This sparks a patient with an unknown illegal drug in his system to begin yelling at the first patient under the influence. Neither patient is capable of rational responses limiting how far they will go because they are not attuned to their surroundings or the consequences of their behavior. After the verbal altercation, both indi-viduals stand up and approach one another. If no one intervenes, a potentially violent situation may occur. The triage nurse needs to rec-ognize what is occurring, call for assistance to defuse the situation, and strive to provide a safe environment for everyone.

SECURITY

Security is utilized in different ways within medical facilities world-wide and includes:

- Weapon-carrying officers employed by or contracted with the facility
- Security guards trained in de-escalation techniques (these guards do not carry weapons)
- Officers or security guards who may be regularly stationed in the area or nearby; at times a phone call is necessary to alert these guards to the need for additional assistance
- Metal detectors or wands used upon entry to the facility to ensure the safety of patients and staff

Smaller facilities, due to lack of resources, may rely on their employees to act as security. Whatever the case may be in your facility, the importance of having well-trained security or other staff available to work with the medical team is critical to minimize the chance of a violent situation occurring.

INCREASING SAFETY IN THE TRIAGE AREA

Measures to increase safety in the triage area are important to ensure that a secure environment is provided for patients, visitors, and staff. Some changes are costly while others have a minimal effect on the budget.

Changes to Make an Area Safe

- Increase lighting in dark areas
- Always have an exit route plan
- Provide all visitors with a name tag stating the room they are visiting; this practice discourages visitors from wandering the department and encourages staff to play an active role in recognizing who belongs where
- Enclose the triage area (e.g., with bullet-resistant glass)
- Install hidden panic buttons that staff can press to alert security or deliver a coded overhead page
- Install closed circuit cameras or video recording
- Provide security attendants when needed
- Provide training for staff in managing aggressive behavior (MOAB) and interpersonal communication

KEEPING THE TRIAGE NURSE AND OTHERS SAFE

The triage nurse's ability to communicate effectively plays a strong role in his or her ability to keep patients and visitors from becoming anxious or confrontational, and in reducing the likelihood that these heightened emotional responses will escalate to agitation or ultimately explode into violence.

Techniques to Keep Safe

- Active listening can help alleviate a patient's or visitor's anxiety and convey a feeling of reassurance. By listening to an individual's concerns the nurse also demonstrates that he or she cares for the individual's well-being

- Be aware of your nonverbal communication; these behaviors and cues express 80% of what you are communicating
  - Leaning forward shows interest in what the patient is saying
  - Standing or sitting at the same level as the patient or visitor helps create a connection between you and the individual
  - Placing your hands by your side rather than folded across the chest expresses a feeling of openness
  - Using "I" statements, such as "I understand what you are saying," provides a reassuring and nonaccusatory response to the individual
  - Using eye contact with your head at an angle rather than straight on appears less confrontational
  - Speaking in a normal tone even if the patient is yelling can help diffuse the situation
- Keep your promise; if you say you will be back in a minute, follow through
- Keep patients updated; lack of information can increase anxiety and frustration

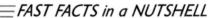 *FAST FACTS in a NUTSHELL*

Being honest and truthful conveys a feeling of caring in an environment that is dynamic and sometimes chaotic.

Case Studies

Anna Sivo Montejano and Lynn Sayre Visser

> *Everybody has a story, scenario, or case study they can share regarding their experiences in a clinic, an emergency department (ED), or as a medic or flight nurse. Articles, books, and magazines can increase a person's knowledge regarding disease processes, peculiar lab results, and unusual imaging findings. However, real-life experiences are what most people never forget. No need to memorize or think of a mnemonic, your remembrance is enough. Cases like these make you think, "Wow, I am happy I learned that!" The following case studies could occur in any department and anywhere. This chapter provides scenarios that will raise your awareness of some high-risk, low-frequency situations.*

Upon conclusion in this chapter, you will be able to:

1. State why you should never disclose to outside sources that an inmate is located within your department
2. List one important precursor to a catastrophic event in an infant
3. Identify one observation that may lead you to suspect domestic violence

CASE STUDIES

Inmate

Caring for inmates in our ED was common. They came in handcuffed, escorted by police, the sheriff, or a correctional officer and as long as they were cuffed and the escort was present, the staff felt safe. Then one day the ED phone rang and the person on the line asked for a patient by name. Not thinking much about it I said, "Oh yes, that patient is here, do you want to talk to him?" The person hung up.

I thought to myself, "That was kind of rude." I approached the officer to let him know that someone had called asking for this inmate. His face went pale. At first I did not realize what I had done. I assumed the caller was another officer or the jail calling. Before I knew it, the officer was making multiple phone calls and requesting that the patient be admitted to the hospital as soon as possible. Only then did I realize the dangerous situation I had created for each individual within the department. When an inmate is no longer in a secured area with electric locked gates, officers, and continuous surveillance, the inmate becomes a prime target to either escape with the help of his friends or be eliminated with the help of his enemies. Remember: One must *never* disclose to outside sources that an inmate is in the facility. Sharing this information can potentially put the officers, staff, and inmate at risk.

Suicidal Patient

A patient presented to triage stating he had a cut on his arm. He appeared unfazed by the injury and spoke in a monotone voice. The patient was asked how the injury occurred, and he simply stated that he cut himself. The nurse proceeded to ask, "What did you cut yourself with?" He pulled out a scalpel and laid it on the counter, and to the nurse's surprise the scalpel was from the facility's ED. The patient was immediately escorted to a private area for further questioning, and the nurse inquired if he had anything else with which he could harm himself. He calmly removed a knife with an 8-inch blade from his pocket. No further injury occurred to the patient and everyone was safe within the ED. Remember: By asking appropriate questions and remaining calm, the triage nurse can play a big role in safe outcomes.

Feeling Funny

Sometimes patients describe symptoms that do not seem to make sense or easily fit into any acuity category, but intuition leads us to make the right decision. A 60-year-old woman arrived to triage with vague complaints of not feeling well, ringing in her ears, and a funny feeling in her chest. She had an irregular heartbeat, 76 beats per minute, blood pressure 122/70, respiratory rate 18, and was afebrile. Nothing else was mentioned in her past medical history besides atrial fibrillation. The nurse assigned this patient a higher acuity level. Initially the patient was stable in her ED bed, but after 1.5 hours there was much commotion in her room. When asked what the ruckus was about, the bedside nurse showed the triage nurse the patient's cardiac rhythm strip, with *4-second pauses*. The "funny feeling in her chest" now made a lot of sense. Remember: Connecting the dots between the patient's chief complaint and signs and symptoms is a critical role of the triage nurse. Always pay attention to subtle clues while triaging.

Diarrhea

An unkempt homeless female patient arrived via ambulance complaining of diarrhea and abdominal pain. No rooms were available within the department. Triage did not seem like a good option due to her intermittent loud cries and her inability to sit in a chair; she was placed on a hallway gurney. She was immediately assessed with the usual questions for a female in her 40s with abdominal pain. The patient's answers raised no immediate concerns for the nurse. Throughout the next hour the patient repeatedly climbed off the gurney and walked, leaning forward toward the bathroom. When questioned about her outbursts, she simply said she was having diarrhea and did not feel well. As the nurses scurried about caring for their heavy patient loads, one nurse noticed that the patient's cries of pain seemed almost rhythmic. A few more questions were asked about her last menstrual cycle, the possibility of pregnancy, vaginal bleeding, and so on. The patient adamantly stated there was no chance of pregnancy because she was currently on her period and had not "done it in years!" Just as the patient began to scream, the nurse lifted up the sheet. The head of a lifeless, blue-faced baby was protruding between the patient's legs. Quickly the staff intervened, successfully resuscitating the baby. Remember: Never let your guard down, because the chance to save a life may be just around the corner.

Newborn Not Eating

A neonate was brought to triage by her parents with a report of poor feeding and excessive sleeping. The triage nurse's first thought was "a newborn sleeping a lot is completely normal!" The new parents appeared anxious. Reassurance was given and they decided to go home, feeling silly for overreacting. The following day, the baby continued to eat poorly and appeared listless, so the worried parents returned to the ED. Upon arrival, the triage nurse removed the blanket covering the baby carrier and discovered the neonate in respiratory arrest. The ED staff successfully resuscitated the baby and a medical workup was completed. The final diagnosis was sepsis. Remember: Assessing each patient visually upon arrival is a must, and often the only symptoms stated by parents prior to a catastrophic event are vague in nature, such as "poor feeding" or "something is just not right."

Foot Pain

A woman in her 40s approached the triage check-in. A man with two children in a stroller stood behind her as the nurse inquired about what was wrong. "I hurt my foot," she replied. The nurse looked down to see the woman wearing flip flops. The top of her left foot was discolored and twice the size of the right foot. When the triage nurse asked what had happened, the woman reported, "I tripped." The nurse looked more closely at the foot but could not imagine how a trip and fall injury could cause the degree of swelling and discoloration that had occurred. She noted that the man stayed close to the woman throughout the triage assessment and often spoke for her. Feeling uneasy with the story, the triage nurse realized she needed a moment alone with the patient to ask further questions. When a technician came to take the woman for a foot x-ray, the triage nurse knew this was her opportunity to further inquire about the injury, so she escorted the patient to radiology. In a concerned tone, the nurse asked the patient if she had been assaulted, which the patient adamantly denied. The nurse gently expressed concern that the injury looked like a crush injury from someone or something stomping on her foot. "You do not need to tell me what happened, but I need you to know that I'm concerned for you," the nurse said. During that short encounter the triage nurse provided the patient with an orthopedic business card. The card was not intended for orthopedic follow up but rather had the number for the organization Women Escaping a Violent Environment, also known as WEAVE. At triage the patient's story does not always match the clinical findings. When this occurs, going the extra mile to ask further questions is a must. Remember: Intimate partner violence is a real concern. Your actions could potentially help or save the life of a person at risk.

FAST FACTS in a NUTSHELL

Despite busy shifts in triage, always stop long enough to make eye contact with your patients, *listen* to their concerns, *look* at their area of complaint, and incorporate *touch* into your assessment. *Compassionate care* and *compassionate actions* go a long way with patients and visitors.

Abbreviations

ABCDE	airway, breathing, circulation, disability, environment/exposure	DTaP	diphtheria, tetanus, and pertussis
ACS	acute coronary syndrome	ECG	electrocardiogram
ALOC	altered level of consciousness	ED	emergency department
		EMC	emergency medical condition
AMA	against medical advice	EMR	electronic medical record
AMI	acute myocardial infarction	EMTALA	Emergency Medical Treatment and Active Labor Act
ASA	acetylsalicylic acid		
ATP	advanced triage protocol	ENA	Emergency Nurses Association
ATS	Australasian Triage Scale		
AVPU	alert, verbal, pain, unresponsive	ESI	Emergency Severity Index
		GCS	Glasgow Coma Scale
BM	bowel movement	GPS	global positioning system
BNP	B-type natriuretic peptide	HCG	human chorionic gonadotropin
bpm	beats per minute		
C&S	culture and sensitivity	HELLP	hemolysis, elevated liver enzyme levels, and low platelet levels
CBC	complete blood count		
CDC	Centers for Disease Control and Prevention		
		HIPAA	Health Insurance Portability and Accountability Act
CMP	complete metabolic panel		
CMS	Centers for Medicare and Medicaid Services		
		HIV	human immunodeficiency virus
COBRA	Consolidated Omnibus Reconciliation Act		
		HT	human trafficking
COPD	chronic obstructive pulmonary disease	ICD	implanted cardioverter defibrillator
		ICU	intensive care unit
CPK	creatinine phosphokinase	INR	international normalized ratio
CPR	cardiopulmonary resuscitation		
		IPV	intimate partner violence
CSE	commercial sexual exploitation		
		L	liter
CST	child sex trafficking	LBTC	left before treatment completed
CT	computed tomography		
CTAS	Canadian Triage Acuity Scale	LOS	length of stay
		LPMSE	left prior to medical screening exam
CXR	chest x-ray		
DKA	diabetic ketoacidosis		

LVAD	left ventricular assist device
LWBS	left without being seen
LWT	left without treatment
MAP	mean arterial pressure
MD	medical doctor
mg/dL	milligrams per deciliter
MI	myocardial infarction
mL	milliliter
mmHg	millimeter of mercury
mmol/L	millimoles per liter
MMR	measles, mumps, and rubella
MOAB	management of aggressive behavior
MSE	medical screening exam
MTS	Manchester Triage System
NIHSS	National Institutes of Health Stroke Scale
NINDS	National Institutes of Neurological Disorders and Stroke
NPO	nothing by mouth
NSAID	nonsteroidal anti-inflammatory drug
PAT	Pediatric Assessment Triangle
PCV	pneumococcal vaccine
pH	potential hydrogen
PHI	personal health information
PID	pelvic inflammatory disease
PMH	past medical history
PQRST	provokes and palliates; quality; region and radiation; severity and associated symptoms; timing and temporal relations

PT	prothrombin time
PTT	partial thromboplastin time
QMP	qualified medical person
Rh	rhesus
RICE	rest, ice, compression, and elevation
RMC	retail medical clinic
RSV	respiratory syncytial virus
r-tPA	tissue plasminogen activator
SBP	systolic blood pressure
SIRS	systemic inflammatory response syndrome
STD	sexually transmitted disease
STEMI	ST-segment elevation myocardial infarction
TDD	telecommunication device for the deaf
TIA	transient ischemic attack
TTD	text-telephone device
UA	urinalysis
UCC	urgent care center
US	ultrasound
VAD	ventricular assist device
WBC	white blood cell count
WR	waiting room
°C	degrees Celsius
°F	degrees Fahrenheit
<	less than
>	greater than
%	percent

Resources

FORMALIZED TRIAGE EDUCATION

- Emergency Nurses Association has online triage education modules available at www.ena.org
- Triage First, Inc. offers both online and live triage education opportunities at www.triagefirst.com
- Health Resources Unlimited, Inc. has online and live education accessible through http://www.hru.net/
- Emergency Department Triage Assessment Course (EDTAC)
- Emergency Triage Assessment and Treatment (ETAT) course
- 2011 Guidelines for Field Triage of Injured Patients Course for EMS Professionals

BOOKS

Several books that may further enhance your triage knowledge base are included in the Additional Reading section. See, in particular, Briggs (2011), Briggs and Grossman (2006), Buettner (2013), Edwards (2013), Emergency Nurses Association (2007, 2009, 2010, 2012, 2013), Manchester Triage Group (2014), Rutenberg and Greenberg (2012), and Zimmermann and Herr (2006).

WEBSITES

Additional triage knowledge can be gained from the following websites:

- http://www.ahrq.gov (access to a free download of the Emergency Severity Index 4th edition training)
- http://caep.ca/resources/ctas (Canadian Triage Acuity Scale [CTAS] resource links and information about mobile device application purchases)
- http://www.who.int (Emergency Triage Assessment and Treatment [ETAT] course manual for participants printed in English and French)
- http://www.health.gov (Australian Government Department of Health and Ageing Emergency Triage Education Kit)
- http://prneducation.ca (CTAS links, with information in English and French)

Additional Reading

Agency for Healthcare Research. (2013). *Team triage reduces emergency depart-ment walkouts, improves patient care*. Retrieved from http://www.innovations .ahrq.gov

American Association for the Surgery of Trauma. (2013). *Trauma facts*. Retrieved from http://www.aast.org

American College of Emergency Physicians. (2013). Meaningful use clarification for emergency department measures. Retrieved from http://www.acep.org/ Advocacy/Meaningful-Use-Clarification-for-Emergency-Department-Measures

American College of Surgeons. (2008). *ATLS manual* (8th ed.). Chicago, IL: Author.

American Heart Association. (2012). *Stroke fact sheet*. Retrieved from http:// www.heart.org

Amsterdam, E. A., Wenger, N. K., Brindis, R. G., Casey, D. E., Jr., Ganiats, T. G., Holmes, D. R., Jr., . . . Zieman, S. J. (2014). 2014 AHA/ACC guide-line for the management of patients with non-ST-elevation acute coronary syndromes: Executive summary: A report of the American College of Cardiology/American Heart Association Task Force on Practice Guidelines. *Circulation, 130*(25), 2354–2394. doi: 10.1161/CIR.0000000000000133.

Anaya, D., & Dellinger, E. P. (2014). Necrotizing soft-tissue infection. *Clinical Infectious Diseases, 44*(5), 705–710.

Aston, J., Bull, N., Gschwandtner, U., Pflueger, M., Borgwardt, S., Stieglitz, R., & Riecher-Rössler, A. (2012). First self-perceived signs and symptoms in emerging psychosis compared with depression. *Early Intervention in Psychiatry, 6*(4), 455–459. doi:10.1111/j.1751-7893.2012.00354.x

Austin, S. (2006). "Ladies & gentlemen of the jury, I present . . . the nursing documentation." *Nursing2006, 36*(1), 56–62.

Australian Government Department of Health. (2009). Emergency triage edu-cation kit. Retrieved May 9, 2014, from http://www.health.gov.au

Baker, S. (2009). *Excellence in the emergency department: How to get results*. Gulf Breeze, FL: Firestarter.

Balentine, J. R., & Davis, C. P. (2013). Human bites. Retrieved September 15, 2014, from http://www.emedicinehealth.com/human_bites/article_ em.htm

Barbee, G., Berry-Caban, C., Daymude, M., Oliver, J., Gay, S. (2012). The ef-fect of provider level triage in a military treatment facility emergency de-partment. *Australasian Journal of Paramedicine, 8*(4). Retrieved from http:// ro.ecu.au/jephc/vol8/iss4/2

Becher, J., & Visovsky, C. (2012). Horizontal violence in nursing, *MedSurg Nursing, 21*(4), 210.

Bemis, P. A. (2011). *Emergency nursing bible* (5th ed.). Huntington Beach, CA: National Nurses in Business Association.

Beveridge, R., Clarke, B., Janes, L., Savage, N., Thompson, J., Dodd, G... Vadeboncoeur, A. (1998). *Implementation guidelines for the Canadian emergency department triage and acuity scale.* Retrieved March 30, 2015, from http://caep.ca/sites/caep.ca/files/caep/files/ctased16.pdf

Billings, D. M., & Halstead, J. A. (2009). *Teaching in nursing: A guide for faculty* (3rd ed.). St. Louis, MO: Elsevier Saunders.

Blair, P. L. (2013). Lateral violence in nursing. *Journal of Emergency Nursing,* 39(5), e75.

Blumberg, P. (2009). *Developing learner-centered teaching: A practical guide for faculty.* San Francisco, CA: Jossey-Bass.

Board of Certification for Emergency Nursing (BCEN). (2009). Value & benefits: Benefits of BCEN certification. Retrieved from http://www.ena .org/bcen/exams/Benefit/Pages/default.aspx

Boxer, B. A., & Boxer Goldfarb, E. M. (2009). The expectations and perceptions of ED patients. *Journal of Emergency Nursing, 35,* 540–541.

Briggs J. K. (2011). *Telephone triage protocols for nurses* (4th ed.). Philadelphia, PA: Lippincott.

Briggs, J., & Grossman, V. (2006). *Emergency nursing: 5-tier triage protocols.* Philadelphia, PA: Lippincott Williams & Wilkins.

Buettner, J. (2013). *Fast facts for the ER nurse: Emergency room orientation in a nutshell* (2nd ed.). New York, NY: Springer Publishing.

Bullard, M., Unger, B., Spence, J., Grafstein, E., & The CTAS National Working Group. (2008). Revisions to the Canadian emergency department triage and acuity. *Canadian Journal of Emergency Medicine, 10*(2), 136–142. doi: 10.2310/8000.2014.012014

Campbell, J. (2012). *International trauma life support* (6th ed.). Boston, MA: Pearson.

Canadian Association of Emergency Physicians. (n.d.). *Canadian triage and acuity scale.* Retrieved from http://caep.ca/resources/ctas#support

Canadian Emergency Department Triage and Acuity Scale Implementation Guidelines. (1999). *Journal Canadian Association Emergency Physician, 2,* 3.

Castner, J., Grinslade, S., Guay, J., Hettinger, A. Z., Seo, J. Y., & Boris, L. (2013). Registered nurse scope of practice and ED complaint-specific protocols. *Journal of Emergency Nursing, 39,* 467–473. doi:10.1016/j.jen.2013.02.009

Center for Emergency Medicine Board Review. (2014). 19th annual The National Emergency Medicine Board Review course. Retrieved from http:// www.ccme.org/nembr

Centers for Disease Control and Prevention. (n.d.). Guidance for the selection and use of personal protective equipment (PPE) in healthcare settings. Retrieved July 23, 2014, from www.cdc.gov

Centers for Disease Control and Prevention. (2009). Transmission of measles. Retrieved June 20, 2014, from www.cdc.gov

Centers for Disease Control and Prevention. (2010). Smallpox basics. Retrieved June 5, 2014, from www.cdc.gov

Centers for Disease Control and Prevention. (2011). National hospital ambulatory medical care survey: 2010 emergency department summary tables. Retrieved February 1, 2014, from http://www.cdc.gov/nchs/data/ahcd/ nhamcs_emergency/2010_ed_web_tables.pdf

Centers for Medicare & Medicaid Services. (2013a). Meaningful use. Retrieved from http://www.cms.gov/Regulations-and-Guidance/Legislation/EHRIncentive Programs/Meaningful_Use.html

Centers for Disease Control and Prevention. (2013b). Parasites—lice. Retrieved June 5, 2014, from www.cdc.gov

Centers for Disease Control and Prevention. (2014a). Immunization schedule for infants and children. Retrieved June 20, 2014, from www.cdc.gov

Centers for Disease Control and Prevention. (2014b). Infection control and prevention. Retrieved July 16, 2014, from www.cdc.gov

Ciocco, M. (2013). *Fast facts for the medical–surgical nurse: Clinical orientation in a nutshell.* New York, NY: Springer Publishing.

Colobong, J. V. & Watson, A. S. (2014). Caring for the patient with acute brain or cranial nerve disorder. In K. S. Osborn, C. E. Wraa, A. S. Watson, & R. S. Holleran (Eds.). *Medical surgical nursing: Preparation for practice* (2nd ed., pp. 503–551) Englewood Cliffs, NJ: Pearson/Prentice-Hall.

Considine, J., Lucas, E., Martin, R., Stergiou, H. E., Kropman, M., & Chiu, H. (2012). Rapid intervention and treatment zone: Redesigning nursing services to meet increasing emergency department demand. *International Journal of Nursing Practice, 18,* 60–67. doi:10.1111/j.1440-172X.2011.01986.x

Convoy, S., & Westphal, R. J. (2013). The importance of developing military cultural competence. *Journal of Emergency Nursing, 39*(6), 591–594. doi:10.1016/j.jen.2013.08.010

Cox, B. (2008). The principles of neurological assessment. *Practice Nurse, 36*(7), 45–50.

Cox, S., Smith, Currell, A., Harriss, L., Barger, B., & Cameron, P. (2011). Differentiation of confirmed major trauma patients and potential major trauma patients using pre-hospital triage criteria. *Injury, 42,* 889–895.

Cushing, T. A., & Alcock, J. (2014) Electrical injuries in emergency medicine clinical presentation. Retrieved October 9, 2014, from http://emedicine .medscape.com/article/770179-clinical

Daniels, R. (2011). Surviving the first hours in sepsis: Getting the basics right (an intensivist's perspective). *Antimicrobial Chemotherapy, 66*(2), ii11–ii23. doi: 10.1093/jac/dkq515

Dateo, J. (2013). What factors increase the accuracy and inter-rater reliability of the emergency severity index among emergency nurses in triaging adult patients? *Journal of Emergency Nursing, 39*(2), 203–207. doi:10.1016/ j.jen.2011.09.002

Day, T., Al-Roubaie, A., Goldlust, E. (2013). Decreased length of stay after addition of healthcare provider in emergency department triage. *Emergency Medicine Journal, 30*(2), 134–138.

DeLemos, C., & Watson, A. S. (2014). Caring for the patient with cerebral vascular disorders. In K. S. Osborn, C. E. Wraa, A. S. Watson, & R. S. Holleran (Eds). *Medical surgical nursing: Preparation for practice* (2nd ed., pp. 552–588). Englewood Cliffs, NJ: Pearson/Prentice-Hall.

Dellinger R., Levy, M., Rhodes, A., Djillali, A., Gerlach, H., Opal, S . . . Surviving Sepsis Campaign Guidelines Committee Including the Pediatric Subgroup. (2013). Surviving sepsis campaign: International guidelines for management of severe sepsis and septic shock. *Critical Care Medicine, 41,* 580–637.

Doerr, S., & Shiel, W. C., Jr. (2014). Heat-related illness. Retrieved October 9, 2014, from http://www.medicinenet.com/hyperthermia/article.htm

Drendel, A., Brousseau, D., & Gorelick, M. (2006). Pain assessment for pediatric patients in the emergency department. *Pediatrics, 117*(5), 1511–1518.

Ducharme, J. (2005). The future of pain management in emergency medicine. *Emergency Medicine Clinics of North America, 23*, 467–475.

Edwards, T. (2013). *The art of triage.* Hauppauge, NY: Nova Science Publishers.

Emergency Nurses Association. (2001). *Making the right decision: A triage curriculum.* (2nd ed.). Des Plaines, IA: Author.

Emergency Nurses Association. (2004). *Course in advanced trauma nursing II: A conceptual approach.* Des Plaines, IL: Author.

Emergency Nurses Association. (2007). *Emergency nursing core curriculum* (6th ed.). St. Louis, MO: Saunders.

Emergency Nurses Association. (2009). *Core curriculum for pediatric emergency nursing* (2nd ed.). Des Plaines, IA: Author.

Emergency Nurses Association. (2010a). Patient satisfaction and customer service in the emergency department. Retrieved October 16, 2014, from www.ena.org

Emergency Nurses Association. (2010b). *Sheehy's emergency nursing principles and practice* (6th ed.). St. Louis, MO: Mosby.

Emergency Nurses Association. (2011). Emergency registered nurse orientation position statement. Retrieved July 18, 2014, from http://www.ena.org

Emergency Nurses Association. (2012a). *Emergency nursing pediatric course: Provider manual* (4th ed.). Des Plaines, IA: Author.

Emergency Nurses Association. (2012b). Geriatric emergency nursing education triage and assessment course. Retrieved on June 29, 2014, from http://www.ena.org

Emergency Nurses Association. (2012c). Specialty certifications in emergency nursing position statement. Retrieved October 16, 2014, from www.ena.org

Emergency Nurses Association. (2013). *Sheehy's manual of emergency care* (7th ed.). St. Louis, MO: Mosby.

Emergency Nurses Association. (2014a). *Trauma nursing core course* (7th ed.). Des Plaines, IA: Author.

Emergency Nurses Association. (2014b). Use of protocols in the emergency setting. Retrieved from https://www.ena.org/SiteCollectionDocuments/Position%20Statements/UseofProtocols.pdf

Evans, H., Summers, R., & Thompson, J. (2011). Implementing scripting in the emergency department: Does it measure up? *Annals of Emergency Medicine, 58*(4), S317. doi: 10.1016/j.annemergmed.2011.06.442

Farrohknia, N., Castren., M., Ehrenberg, A., Lars. L., Oredsson, S., Jonsson, H. . . . Göransson, K. (2011). Emergency department triage scales and their components: A systematic review of the scientific evidence. *Scandinavian Journal of Trauma, Resuscitation & Emergency Medicine, 19*, 42. Retrieved from http://www.sjtrem.com/content/19/1/42

FitzGerald, G., Jelinek, G. A., Scott, D., & Gerdtz, M. F. (2010). Emergency department triage revisited. *Emergency Medicine Journal, 27*, 86–92. doi:10.1136/emj.2009.077081

Flanagan, M. (2005). Every patient deserves a safe nurse. *American Journal of Nursing, 105*(11), 112.

Foley, A. (2011). Talking the talk in triage. *Journal of Emergency Nursing, 37*(2), 205–206. doi: 10.1016/j.jen.2010.11.009

Foley, A., & Durant, J. (2011). Let's ask that out front: Health and safety screening in triage. *Journal of Emergency Nursing, 37*(5), 515.

Fosnocht, D. E., Swanson, E. R., & Barton, E. D. (2005). Changing attitudes about pain and pain control in emergency medicine. *Emergency Medicine Clinics of North America, 23,* 297–306.

Foster, S. C. & Hampton, R. Jr. (2014). Stevens-Johnson syndrome treatment and management. Retrieved March 19, 2015, from http://emedicine .medscape.com/article/1197450-treatment

Galioto, N. (2008). Peritonsillar abscess. *American Family Physician, 77*(2), 199–202.

Gerdtz, M., & Bucknall, T. (1999). Why we do the things we do: Applying clinical decision-making frameworks to triage practice. *Accident and Emergency Nursing, 7*(1), 50–57.

Grossman, V. A. (2014). *Fast facts for the radiology nurse: An orientation and nursing care guide in a nutshell.* New York, NY: Springer Publishing.

Halliday, A. (2005). Creating a reliable time line. *Nursing2005, 35*(2), 27.

Hammond, B. B. (2012). Cardiovascular emergencies. In B. B. Hammond & P. G. Zimmermann (Eds.), *Sheehy's manual of emergency care* (7th ed.). St Louis, MO: Elsevier.

Handel, D., Fu, R., Daya, M., York, J., Larson, E., & McConnell, K. (2010). The use of scripting at triage and its impact on elopements. *Academic Emergency Medicine, 17,* 495–500. doi: 10.1111/j.1553-2712.2010.00721.x

Hayden, C., Burlingame, P., Thompson, H., & Sabol, V. (2013). Improving patient flow in the emergency department by placing a family nurse practitioner in triage: A quality improvement project. *Journal of Emergency Nursing, 40*(4), 346–351. doi: 10.1016/j.jen.2013.09.011

Hohenhaus, S. (2006). Someone watching over me: Observations in pediatric triage. *Journal of Emergency Nursing, 32*(5), 398–403.

Holleran, R. S., & Wraa, C. E. (2014). Caring for the patient with multisystem trauma. In K. S. Osborn, C. E. Wraa, A. S. Watson, & R. S. Holleran (Eds.). *Medical-surgical nursing: Preparation for practice* (2nd ed., pp. 2091–2112). Englewood Cliffs, NJ: Pearson/Prentice-Hall.

Hoyt, K. S., & Selfridge-Thomas, J. (2007). *Emergency nursing core curriculum* (6th ed., pp. 459–460). Philadelphia, PA: Saunders/Elsevier.

Innes, K., Plummer, V., & Considine, V. (2011). Nurses' perceptions of their preparation for triage. *Australasian Emergency Nursing Journal, 14*(2), 81–86.

Janiak, B. D. (2009). Seven ways to succeed in getting sued (without really trying). *ED Legal Letter,* March 1.

The Joint Commission. (2013). *Specifications manual for national hospital inpatient quality measures.* Retrieved from http://www.jointcommission.org

Kothari R. U., Pancioli A., Liu T., Brott T., & Broderick J. (1999). Cincinnati Prehospital Stroke Scale: Reproducibility and validity. *Annals of Emergency Medicine, 33*(4), 373–378.

Kroekel, P. A., George, L., & Eltoukhy, N. (2013). How to manage the patient in the emergency department with a left ventricular assist device. *Journal of Emergency Nursing, 39*(5), 447–453. doi:10.1016/j.jen.2012.01.007

Lavoie-Tremblay, M., Leclerc, E., Marchionni, C., & Drevniok, U. (2010). The needs and expectations of generation Y nurses in the workplace. *Journal for Nurses in Staff Development, 26*(1), 2–8.

Liedtke, B. (2013). The case for mentoring in emergency departments. *Australian College for Emergency Medicine*, 1–12. (version 1.1)

Lombardo, B., & Eyre, C. (2011). Compassion fatigue: A nurse's primer. *Online Journal of Issues in Nursing, 16*(1), 3. doi: 10.3912/OJIN.Vol16No01Man03

Lorenzi, N. M., Kouroubali, A., Detmer, D. E., & Bloomrosen, M. (2009). How to successfully select and implement electronic health records (EHR) in small ambulatory practice settings. *BMC Medical Informatics and Decision Making, 9*, 15–28. doi:10.1186/1472-6947-9-15

Love, R., Murphy, J., Lietz, T., & Jordan, K. (2012). The effectiveness of a provider in triage in the emergency department: A quality of improvement initiative to improve patient flow. *Advanced Emergency Nursing Journal, 34*(1), 65–74. doi: 10.1097/TME.0b013e3182435543

Manchester Triage Group. (2014). *Emergency triage: Manchester triage group* (3rd ed.). Chichester, UK: John Wiley.

Manchester Triage System. (n.d.). Retrieved from http://www.triagenet.net/en

McCarthy, M., Zeger, S., Ding, R., Levin, S., Desmond, J., Lee, J., & Arnosky, D. (2009). Crowding delays treatment and lengthens emergency department length of stay, even among high-acuity patients. *Annals of Emergency Medicine, 54*(4), 492–503.e4.

Morrison, K. J. (2014). *Fast facts for stroke care nursing: An expert guide in a nutshell.* New York, NY: Springer Publishing.

Muller, M. L. (2014). *Pediatric bacterial meningitis clinical presentation.* Retrieved September 15, 2014, from http://emedicine.medscape.com/article/961497-clinical

Murray, M., Bullard, M., & Grafstein, E.; CTAS National Working Group; CEDIS National Working Group. (2004). Revisions to the Canadian Emergency Department Triage and Acuity Scale implementation guidelines. *Canadian Journal of Emergency Medicine, 6*(6), 421–427.

National Institute of Neurological Disorders and Stroke. (2011). Guillain-Barre syndrome fact sheet. NIH Pub. No. 11-2902. Retrieved from http://www.ninds.nih.gov/disorders/gbs/detail_gbs.htm

O'Gara, P. T., Kushner, F. G., Ascheim, D. D., Casey, D. E., Jr., Chung, M. K., de Lemos, J. A., . . . CF/AHA Task Force. (2013). 2013 ACCF/AHA guideline for the management of ST-elevation myocardial infarction: A report of the American College of Cardiology Foundation/American Heart Association Task Force on Practice Guidelines. *Circulation, 127*(4), 529–555. doi: 10.1161/CIR.0b013e3182742c84

Pante, M., & Pollak, A. (Eds.). (2010). *Advanced assessment & treatment of trauma.* Boston, MA: Jones & Bartlett.

Pearson, H. (2013). Science and intuition: Do both have a place in clinical decision making? *British Journal of Nursing, 22*(4), 212–215.

Pich, J., Hazelton M., Sundin, D., & Kable, A., (2011). Patient-related violence at triage: Qualitative descriptive study. *International Emergency Nursing, 19*, 12–19.

Pines, J. M., Hilton, J. A., Weber, E. J., Alkemade, A. J., Al Shabanah, H., Anderson, P. D., . . . Schull, M. J. (2011). International perspectives on emergency department crowding. *Academic Emergency Medicine, 18*, 1358–1370. doi: 10.1111/j.1553-2712.2011.01235.x

Pines, J., & Hollander, J. (2008). Emergency department crowding is associated with poor care for patients with severe pain. *Annals of Emergency Medicine, 51*(1), 1–5.

Press Ganey Associates, Inc. (2009). Pulse report 2009 emergency department patient perspective on American health care. Retrieved from http://www.pressganey.com/galleries/ED_Pulse_2009_files/2009_ED_Pulse_Report.pdf

Randall, J. R., Colman, I., & Rowe, B. H. (2011). A systematic review of psychometric assessment of self-harm risk in the emergency department (Structured abstract). *Journal of Affective Disorders, 134*(1), 348–355. doi:10.1016/j.jad.2011.05.032

Rehberg, S., Maybauer, M., Enkhbaatar, P., Maybauer, D., Yamamoto, Y., & Traber, D. (2010). Pathophysiology, management and treatment of smoke inhalation injury. *Expert Review of Respiratory Medicine, 3*(3), 282–297.

Retezar, R., Bessman, E., Ding, R., Zeger, S. L., & McCarthy, M. L. (2011). The effect of triage diagnostic standing orders on emergency department treatment time. *Annals of Emergency Medicine, 57*(2), 89–99. doi:10.1016/j.annemergmed.2010.05.016

Robinson, D. J. (2013). An integrative review: Triage protocols and the effect on ED length of stay. *Journal of Emergency Nursing, 39*, 398–408. doi:10.1016/j.jen.2011.12.016

Rowe, B. H., Villa-Roel, C., Guo, X., Bullard, M. J., Ospina, M., Vandermeer, B., . . . Holroyd, B. R. (2011). The role of triage nurse ordering on mitigating overcrowding in emergency departments: A systematic review. *Academic Emergency Medicine, 18*, 1349–1357. doi:10.1111/j.1553-2712.2011.01081.x

Russ, S., Jones, I., Aronsky, D., Dittus, R. S., & Slovis, C. M. (2010). Placing physician orders at triage: The effect on length of stay. *Annals of Emergency Medicine, 56*(1), 27–33. doi:10.1016/j.anneemergmed.2010.02.006

Rutenberg, C., & Greenberg, E. (2012). *The art and science of telephone triage: How to practice nursing over the phone.* Hot Springs, AR: Telephone Triage Consulting, Inc.

Sanchez, C., Valdez, A., & Johnson, L. (2014). Hoop dancing to prevent and decrease burnout and compassion fatigue. *Journal of Emergency Nursing, 40*(4), 394.

Smith, E., Saver, J. L., Alexander, D. N., Furie, K. L., Hopkins, L. N., Katzan, I. L., . . . Williams, L. S.; on behalf of the AHA/ASA Stroke Performance Oversight Committee. (2014). Clinical performance measures for adults hospitalized with acute ischemic stroke: Performance measures for healthcare professionals from the American Heart Association/American Stroke Association. *Stroke, 45*(11), 3472–3498. doi: 10.1161/STR.0000000000000045

Stauber, M. A. (2013). Advanced nursing interventions and length of stay in the emergency department. *Journal of Emergency Nursing, 39*, 221–225. doi:10.1016/j.jen.2012.02.015

Studer, Q., Hagins, M., & Cochrane, B. (2014). The power of engagement: Creating the culture that gets your staff aligned and invested. *Healthcare Management Forum, 27*, S79–S87. doi:10.1016/j.hcmf.2014.01.008

Sulfaro, S. (2009). Charting the course for triage decisions. *Journal of Emergency Nursing, 35*(3), 268–269. doi:10.1016/jen.2009.01.003

Svinicki, M., & McKeachie, W. J. (2011). *McKeachie's teaching tips: Strategies, research, and theory for college and university teachers* (13th ed.). Belmont, CA: Wadsworth.

Thoms, K. (2012). They're not just big kids: Motivating adult learners. Retrieved March 18, 2014, from http://frank.mtsu.edu/~itconf/proceed01/22.html

Tintinalli, J. E., Kelen, G. D., & Stapczynski, J. S. (2004). *Emergency medicine: A comprehensive study guide* (6th ed.). New York, NY: McGraw-Hill.

Tipsord-Klinkhammer, B., & Andreoni, C. P. (1998). *Quick reference to emergency nursing*. Philadelphia, PA: W. B. Saunders.

Triage First, Inc. (2013). *ED triage: Comprehensive course*. Asheville, NC: Author.

Triage First, Inc. (2012). *ED triage comprehensive course; ED triage systematics, documentation lecture*. Asheville, NC: Author.

Vartak, S., Crandall, D. K., Brokel, J. M., Wakefield, D. S., & Ward, M. M. (2009). Professional practice and innovation: Transformation of emergency department processes of care with EHR, CPOE, and ER even tracking. *Health Information Management Journal, 38*(2), 27–32.

Vitulano, N., Riccioni, G., & Trivisano, A. (2012). Atypical presentation of acute coronary syndrome–not ST elevation: A case report. *Care Reports in Medicine*, 1–3. doi:10.1155/2012/182379

Warren, D. W., Jarvis, A., Le Blanc, L., Gravel, J., & CTAS National Working Group. (2008). Revisions to the Canadian triage & acuity scale paediatric guidelines (PaedCTAS). *Canadian Journal of Emergency Medicine, 10*(3), 224–232. Retrieved from http://www.cjem-online.ca/v10/n3/p224

Weingarten, R. M., & Weingarten, C. T. (2013). Generational diversity in ED and education settings: A daughter–mother perspective. *Journal of Emergency Nursing, 39*(4), 369–371.

Welch, S. (2008). Preventing ED violence starts in triage. *Emergency Medicine News, 30*(12), 4. doi:10.1097/01.EEM.0000342733.39531.17

Wiler, J., Gentle, C., Halfpenny, J., Heins, A., Mehrotra, A., Mikhail, M., & Fite, D. (2009). Optimizing emergency department front-end operations. *Annals of Emergency Medicine, 55*(2), 142–160. doi: 10.1016/j.annemergmed.2009.05.021

World Health Organization. (2014). Emergency triage assessment and treatment (ETAT) course. Retrieved June 6, 2014, from http://www.who.int

Yang, C. Y., Liu, H. Y., Lin, H. L., & Lin, J. N. (2012). Left-sided acute appendicitis: A pitfall in the emergency department. *Journal of Emergency Medicine, 43*(6), 980–982. doi: 10.1016/j.jemermed.2010.11.056

Zimmermann, P. G., & Herr, R. D. (2006). *Triage nursing secrets*. St Louis, MO: Elsevier.

Index